DE 27 '79

W9-BAV-434

Heidelberg
Science
Library

Heidelberg
Science
Library

Valentino Braitenberg

On the
Texture of Brains

Springer-Verlag
New York
Heidelberg
Berlin

An Introduction
to Neuroanatomy
for the
Cybernetically Minded

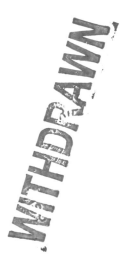
WITHDRAWN

Professor Dr. Valentino Braitenberg
Hon.-Professor, Universität Tübingen;
Hon.-Professor, Universität Freiburg;
Direktor am Max-Planck-Institut
für biologische Kybernetik,
D-7400 Tübingen

Translated into English by Dr. Elisabeth Hanna Braitenberg and by the author.

Title of the original edition: Gehirngespinste. Neuroanatomie für ky-
bernetisch Interessierte. © Springer-Verlag Berlin Heidelberg 1973

Library of Congress Cataloging in Publication Data

Braitenberg, Valentino.
   On the texture of brains.
   (Heidelberg science library)
   Translation of Gehirngespinste.
   Bibliography: p.
   Includes index.
   1. Brain-Anatomy. 2. Cybernetics. I. Title.
II. Series.
QM455.B6513   611'.8   77-21851

All rights reserved
No part of this book may be translated or reproduced in any
form without written permission from Springer-Verlag.
© 1977 Springer-Verlag New York Inc.
Printed in Germany.

987654321

ISBN 0-387-08391-X Springer-Verlag New York Heidelberg Berlin

ISBN 3-540-08391-X Springer-Verlag Berlin Heidelberg New York

QM
455
.B6513

143222

Dedicated

to the taxpayers of three lovable countries who supported our studies*, always waiting patiently for explanations.

* *through the University of Rome, the Deutsche Forschungsgemeinschaft, Yale University, the University of Naples, the Air Force Office of Scientific Research, the National Institutes of Health, the Consiglio Nazionale delle Ricerche, the Max-Planck-Gesellschaft, and the University of Tübingen.*

Thanks

are due to Dr. Campos-Ortega (now Freiburg) for the
negative of Figure 4.4, to Dr. Mayer (Tübingen) for the
silver preparation of Figure 5.5, to the memory of Prof.
Edinger (Frankfurt/Main) for the myelin preparation of
Figure 8.1 and to Prof. Krücke (Frankfurt/Main) for the
loan of the same. The remaining preparations were made
by my exquisite staff of histologists: E. Sada, V. Gugliel-
motti, and E. Casale (Naples) and E. Hartwieg, M. L.
Obermayer, A. Sada, D. Stoll, and K. Witte (Tübingen).
The drawings were prepared by M. L. Obermayer and by
C. Braitenberg, both patient beyond the call of duty.
Special thanks to Miss G. Kurz, M. A., for the painstak-
ing labor of bookkeeping and bookmaking.

Preface

I believe that the most intriguing thing in the world, besides the world itself, is the human brain. Moreover,
I am sure that a coherent natural philosophy will only be
possible once we have understood how the brain, itself
an object of physics, generates the description of the
physical word. Therefore a book on the brain, be it the
fly's or the mouse's brain, needs no justification. It is
important, however, to point out the limits of its ambi-
tions. The first three Chapters are introductory and are
written in a lighthearted philosophical vein. An idea is
introduced that turns up repeatedly in the rest of the
book, namely, that the structure of brains is information
about the world. Chapter 4 is didactic: in it the neuron
and its function are sketched as the element of the nervous tissue. Chapters 5 to 8 are a collection of essays
loosely tied together mainly by the vagaries of my own
interests. They do not intend to be definitive statements
about the cerebellum, the cerebral cortex, or the visual
ganglia of insects but rather illuminate these structures
from a personal point of view. Accordingly, many authors will find their own contributions only insufficiently
represented in the text and frequently without explicit
quotation. I beg their pardon and remind the reader that
enough competent reviews are available in the fields that
I touch upon, easily accessible through the references.
Chapter 7 does not represent the latest phase of the discussion on optomotor reactions in insects which flourish-

es in our institute. I hope with my conservatism to counteract the effect of propinquity and personal involvement: had I accepted all the recommendations that were given to me at the time when I prepared the first (German) edition, I would have been forced to change the text now much more than I had to change my rather conservative essay of a few years ago. New material has been introduced wherever it seemed necessary. The Chapter on information was enlarged by a didactic essay. Chapter 8, on the cerebral cortex, is completely rewritten and incorporates some of our own research since the first edition. As before, it explodes at the end into a burst of speculation that is connected with a contention at the beginning of the book: neuroanatomy, an approach to psychology.

Summer 1977   V. Braitenberg

Contents

1 Neuroanatomy, Psychology, and
Animism   1

2 Physics and Antiphysics   5

3 Information   9

4 What Brains Are Made Of   19

5 How Accurately Are Brains
Designed?   41

6 Neuroanatomical Invariants: Analysis of the
Cerebellar Cortex   59

7 The Automatic Pilot of the Fly   83

8 The Common Sensorium: An Essay on the
Cerebral Cortex   101

Subject Index   123

1. Neuroanatomy, Psychology, and Animism

. . . For to explain has always been to exorcise . . .
Samuel Beckett, Watt [1.1]¹

I want to sell neuroanatomy as a kind of psychology — as its most concrete and ultimate form. This may not be what people have in mind who turn to psychology expecting confirmation of their own insights into conscious and unconscious motivations. Rather, this essay is intended as a contribution to a new science of the mind as it is bound to emerge soon. I am sure that computer science, attempts at creating "artificial intelligence", in short, the techniques of information processing will lead the way.

It is a fact that almost everything that interests us in our dealings with other people can be transmitted without difficulty in the form of electric signals through a wire. The charms of an actress are a pattern of electromagnetic waves in the antenna before they appear on the television screen. I can experience that malicious humor of a friend as intensely over the telephone as I can face to face. The results of a piece of scientific work can be transmitted through a wire, for example, in the form of a telegram. What is remarkable is this: all these rarefied psychological things — charm, maliciousness, intellect, humor — should, in principle, be discoverable in a physical study of the wave pattern in the wire. They should correspond to abstract but precisely describable properties of the variations of the electric potential in the wire. Of course, if one observes the wire instead of the human who generates the information, one may discover complicated formulas far removed from the immediate understanding which we experience in direct personal contact. In principle, however, we can sense that it is possible to deal with psychological phenomena the same way as with those of physics. There is no qualitative difference between the transmission of a simple phenomenon, such as an alternating cur-

---

¹ Numbers in brackets refer to references, which are listed at the end of each chapter.

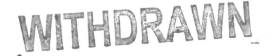
WITHDRAWN

rent, and of something as complicated as the time course of the potential resulting in the humorous remark of my friend at the other end of
the wire, but rather a difference in the level of complexity of these
phenomena.

To be sure, very different machinery will have to be used in order
to recognize the characteristics of the electric phenomena in the wire
at various levels of complexity: one kind of equipment is necessary to
count off series of pulses, and another to determine the frequency of
an alternating current, a very different one again to determine whether or not the number of pulses in a series is a prime number. It is not
easy to say what kind of an apparatus would be necessary to judge the
correctness of grammar in a text transmitted through a teletype system, and we would be completely at a loss if we had to construct
something that was to decide whether the text is serious or humorous.
The hierarchy of complexity is characterized by discrete levels, each
corresponding to a kind of apparatus sufficient for recognizing patterns at that level of complexity. It seems that in some mysterious way
the human brain is still the most powerful machine equipped to
handle patterns at all levels.

We are interested in brains because we hope that by dealing with
the nervous system we will come closer to an understanding of psychology, which is our main concern. Once we have understood how
a brain responds to humor, or how it recognizes the correctness of
grammar, we shall also have better definitions of these abstract concepts.

It may be surprising to some that it is neuroanatomy, rather than
electrophysiology, that I propose to relate to the computer-like
aspects of the brain. Perhaps I should rather say that neuroanatomy
points especially to the brain-like computers of the future. As I hope
to show in the rest of this book, we learn in neuroanatomy how the
spatial coordinates within a brain are used in a meaningful way as an
essential part of the information processing system, a principle which,
as yet, has hardly been incorporated in digital computers. Also, everything in neuroanatomy points toward a diffuse and intimate mixing of
logic and memory, of the processes that determine structure on the
basis of a preordained plan, and of those that modify the structure on
the basis of experience. This, too, is as yet more on the science fiction
side of today's technological development.

Even the results of electrophysiology have done much to strength-
en our faith in the study of brain anatomy. The most fundamental
result of microelectrode recording from single neurons within the living brain is this: one may record totally different signals when one

moves the tip of an electrode by a distance corresponding to the separation of two neighboring neurons within the brain, or, in other words: the complexity that is apparent in the microscopic observation of the tissue is the true complexity of the information that the brain can deal with. Moreover, there is a pessimistic note in microelectrode neurophysiology when one considers that the relevant chunks of experience (things, persons, attitudes, sentences) are most likely not represented within the brain by single neurons, but by sets of neurons too numerous to be observed systematically by means of arrays of microelectrodes. The neuroanatomy of neuronal networks will be for quite some time, and perhaps forever, the context that relates the physiology of single neurons and synapses to the macroscopic events of psychology.

Neuroanatomy is also, in the medical schools, a major part of that monstruous exercise in memorization that the student has to go through at the beginning of his career, perhaps designed to weed out those minds that will be unable, later on, to greet every patient by his name along with a reference to the organ affected. Some of this teaching is probably justified by the importance of neuroanatomy in localizing brain damage on the basis of scattered neurologic symptoms, although in the hands of medical practitioners this reduces to an awesome recollection of the complexity of the nervous system and to the feeling that such patients are best sent to specialized neurologic institutions. I am afraid the medical student will find little help if he turns to this book hoping to find mnemonic aids for the mastery of fiber tracts in the human brain. He may gain the feeling, however, that the whole brain is in its own way a mnemonic device, waiting to be explained as such, and he may begin to exercise his imagination accordingly.

I will not talk about macroscopic anatomy because I feel that it is difficult to deal with the major subdivisions of the brain and with the fiber tracts connecting them without relapsing into an attitude that I am trying to overcome in this book. At the gross anatomical level, the tie between psychology and nervous structure, often called functional neuroanatomy, is a mapping of macroscopic subdivisions of the psyche onto macroscopic subdivisions of the brain. Initiative, for example, is said to be localized in the frontal lobes of the mammalian brain, and rage in the amygdala. If you use this language, you have already implicitly declared that you are not interested in knowing the whole complexity of the situation called "initiative" or "rage", since if you really were, you would feel uneasy with the global psychological terms and would try to define mechanisms instead. You would not rest before you had satisfied yourself that the neuronal wiring of the frontal cortex or that of the amygdala is exactly what it takes to produce the phenomena that are called initiative or rage. To some people, a mechanism is a box that can be used to do certain tricks; to others, it is the springs and levers inside. What we really want to know is how the use is related to the structure.

The idea that psychological complexities can in principle be identified with the structure of a highly organized piece of matter, the human brain, is unappealing to many people. Something in their mental setup balks at the idea that the colorful, lovable experience of themselves and of other persons is translatable into the black and white drawing of a set of logical relations. They would rather leave the psyche unanalyzed and think of it as a separate substance that has a fleeting liaison with the body as long as it lives. This view is called animism when it is encountered by ethnologists in other societies. It is also the most widespread psychological theory in our own society, where it is supported by innumerable amateur researchers and believers in extrasensory perception, transmigration of souls, transcendental meditation etc. It is not possible to prove animism wrong, and there is very little one can show in support of the other view, which would reduce psychological experience to mathematical structure. It is important, however, to realize that the animistic heresy has been competing against the analytic tendency of science throughout the history of philosophy. It turns up even within our own science as the subconscious motive of reports on experiences that can be passed from one animal to another in a filtered extract of the brain, or in the form of defeatist statements about the nature of language, or in such odd conceptual conglomerations as that of the laconic case history that I once discovered in a world-famous department of psychiatry: "the patient has fits during which he loses feces, urine, and consciousness."

References

1.1 Beckett, S.: Watt (Paris 1953), London: Calder and Boyars, 1970

2. Physics and Antiphysics

For a long time it seemed as if in natural science the problem of language played only a secondary rôle.
W. Heisenberg, 1960 [2.1]

There are things that are difficult to recognize, not because they are too small for our eyes, but because they are too complex. In coming to terms with a difficult mathematical treatise or a poem written in a concentrated style, a magnifying glass will not help. Studying the exact form of the letters does not contribute to an understanding of the text. Even if, at the next higher level, we understand the letters as phonemes, and study the statistical laws of their combinations in a certain language, we may learn something about speech mechanisms and the structure of the language, but we will learn nothing about the meaning of the text. A particular text cannot be explained from the rules that govern a language.

This obvious fact has to be mentioned because it is in contrast with a habit of thought we have appropriated from physics, and which we sometimes use uncritically. Physicists tend to explain the variety of forms at the macroscopic level, i. e., at the level to which our observation has direct access, by descending to the next lower level where particles are discovered or postulated that escape macroscopic observation. If the postulated or observed interactions of the particles lead to theoretical constructs from which the macroscopically observed forms can be derived, then this is taken as the explanation of the macroscopic level. The shape of crystals is explained as a consequence of the geometry of the orderly network resulting from the interactions of neighboring atoms.

I maintain that in studying brains, the strategy to adopt has more to do with the study of a text than with the analysis of a physical observation.

Just as all of literature consists of strings of letters taken from an alphabet of about 30 signs, the same for all texts in a certain language, the hundreds of thousands of different animal brains (the number of animal species that have a brain comes close to one million) consist of different combinations of very few cell types: neurons, glia cells, and some other elements concerned with the delivery and disposal of metabolic products (in blood vessels and tracheoles and in the membranes enveloping the nerve tissue). It may even be argued that nothing is lost if we describe brains only in terms of neurons. These "particles" are found with surprising uniformity in all brains. The uniformity is in their fine structure, the electrochemical properties of their cell membrane, the way they conduct signals and transmit them to other neurons. The variation is, rather, in the form and size of the fibrous cell processes with which they touch each other. The species-specific and individual blueprint of a brain is written in the language of the geometric relations of the neuronal cell processes. The particular tasks that one brain can accomplish, the peculiarities that distinguish the behavior of one animal from that of another, must be principally due to differences in the connective scheme and not in the characteristics of single cells.

From this we may conclude that a specific brain cannot be explained from the general properties of neurons just as a particular text cannot be explained by starting with the transition probabilities of the letters in texts of a certain language. The transition probabilities in the case of the neurons correspond to the average distribution of their cell processes around the cell body; in the same analogy a particular word in the text corresponds to a particular scheme of the connections between the neurons.

Even the question as to what types of brains are at all possible, and what brains are certainly impossible, can only be given a very vague answer on the basis of what we know about single neurons. Barring grotesque fantasies, we come closest to the truth by saying: everything thinkable is possible. Some neurons are found making connections over a distance equaling the diameter of the whole animal, while others are connected only to their nearest neighbors. A neuron can transmit its signals to just one other neuron or to many thousands. The signal transmitted from one neuron to another may be only a very small fraction of the excitation that causes the neuron to become active, or it alone may be enough. Above all, there seem to be all shades of possibilities ranging from an apparently purely statistical distribution of cell processes, not more regular than the distribution of branches on a tree, to very precise patterns of connections of neurons among each other. In other words, the language in which brains are written is a very free language. We will not be able, in most cases, to explain the peculiarities of a certain brain structure by invoking the rules and constraints of the mechanisms that synthesize brains out of neurons, but will always have to consider explanations in terms of the function it performs.

The distinction between crystals and texts, between objects that are explained at the level of the particles out of which they are composed, and those whose explanation lies in a context encompassing the objects themselves (as for example, the explanation of a statement from the social context between the speaker and listener) may seem artificial and unnecessary. It is certainly true that both kinds of explanations have something in common, namely, the extension of the observation, either in the microscopic or the macroscopic direction, until the enlarged field of view allows for the recognition of structures and regularities that were previously hidden. It is a question of taste whether or not we wish to see a profound philosophical polarity in the distinction between the two kinds of explanations or, in connection with this, between several kinds of causality. I would merely like to point out that the two kinds of explanations make different strategies necessary and create different general attitudes toward science. The discipline that is sometimes called cybernetics is the field in which both kinds of explanations are legitimately at home, causal explanations as well as explanations from the context. It is also the science of information carriers, or the science of complex things, which is another way of saying the same thing.

Complexity, roughly, is measured by the number of elements of a situation that I have to mention in order to explain a macroscopic phenomenon. Here it is important to distinguish between the mention of a set of things and the mention of the individual things. An example of the first case is if we explain the pressure of a gas by the movement of individual molecules in the container. Although we are talking about a large number of particles, we are considering them statistically. As far as our consideration goes, they are interchangeable; only the molecules in a collective sense are of interest, not the fate of single molecules. Although the gas represents a complicated situation and although the formulas of statistical mechanics that enable us to derive the pressure of the gas from the movement of molecules may look very complicated, I would like to reserve the word "complex" (as distinct from "complicated") for another kind of situation.

A piece of skin from a stranger that is transplanted in place of my own releases reactions that result in a rejection of the transplant. Only my twin brother's skin can be grafted onto my body without difficulty. The difference can only be explained by detailed reference to the text written as an orderly sequence of submolecules within the thread-like giant molecules. This is apparently variable from individual to individual. Such giant molecules are truly complex: the statistical description misses the point. In order to account for the peculiar affinity between the substance of my twin brother and my own, I cannot avoid a detailed mention of a very large number of individual units.

Perception is also complex. I recognize someone whom I last saw twenty years ago. The rhythm of his walk plays a part in this, the way his hair curls, the style of speech he uses in expressing himself, perhaps the odor of his tobacco or his clothes. The perception of this person is a complex affair and demands a complex brain: it is not a simple, one-dimensional measurement that is involved here, neither his weight, his size, the color of his hair, nor any such simple quantity, but a small region in the multidimensional space of my perception in which only he fits.

At the very root of the distinction between the objects of physics and those of biology we observe that the latter are essentially the result of (genetic or individual) memory processes. A physicist, or a biophysicist for that matter, will always try as best he can to isolate the things he is studying from the accidental environment in which he performs his experiment. He is interested in those properties of matter that are repeatably the same whether he measures them here and now, or later somewhere else. On the contrary, when we talk about the brain of the frog, about the behavior of white American housewives, or about the markings on a butterfly's wings, we are dealing with things that are essentially historical, not invariant in time and space, and therefore not to be considered in isolation from their environment. Living matter is in a very fundamental sense always an image of the world.

I hope these remarks will convince the reader that the antithesis mentioned in the title of this chapter does not reflect any antipathy toward the most beautiful of sciences, but rather an invitation to extend its canons and morals even to fields which, at first sight, seem to go in a direction opposite to that of traditional physics, such as the kind of interpretative neuroanatomy that I am proposing here.

References

2.1 Heisenberg, W.: Sprache und Wirklichkeit in der modernen Physik (1960). In: Schritte über Grenzen, gesammelte Reden und Aufsätze. München: Piper & Co., 1971

3. Information

Out of metaphysical tits
drivel the bits?
Is it a finger without a hand
that writes in the sand of my brain?
A hand without an arm,
an arm without a brain,
or a brain without a soul?
                    (from a German popular song)

... things arise and perish only by composition and
separation, and there is no other arising and perish-
ing, but they abide eternal.   *Anaxagoras [3.1]*

Through visible things we see the invisible ones.
                              Anaxagoras [3.1]

We have already accustomed ourselves to the idea that the study of a brain as an information processing device is more comparable to reading a text than to the causal analysis of an experiment in physics.

But if this is so, who wrote the text? Does it make sense to talk about information when its generator in the form of a talking creature is missing? Can we speak of information where forms have arisen by chance? According to the theory of evolution, are not the structures of animal bodies simply the passive result of a long chain of chance variations accompanied by changes of the probability of survival from one generation to another?

We shall consider a few contexts in which the concept of information is used.

1. A television screen produces about a million bits per second. This is the original context [3.3]. The measure of information, here as a flow of information in bits per second, comes from engineering where the question was: how can pictures or texts that are present in one location be reproduced in another? In this context it is irrelevant who originally produced the information, what it means, or how much of it will be understood. The question is, rather, of how many single

units must an information carrier (a channel) consist in order to hold (or transmit) a certain amount of information. If the information carrier is a mosaic made of black and white tiles of equal size, then the number of tiles I need in order to present a recognizable image is a measure (in bits) of the information content of the original picture. If I figure out how long it takes to rearrange the tiles until I get another picture, I will also know how many bits per second my information carrier can handle (channel capacity).

2. A waking person, e. g., one sitting in front of a television screen, can process between 10 and 20 bits per second. Here man himself becomes a "channel". The information capacity, originally a measure of the mobility of the channel interposed between the transmitter and the receiver, is here applied to the subject of a psychological experiment who has been inserted between the input and output of the experiment and who is instructed to press different keys in answer to different stimuli, or who sight-reads music as fast as he can, etc. One is astonished when one compares the million bits-per-second of the television screen with the 20 bits-per-second that humans can digest, especially since the television consumer immediately has his set repaired if it does not produce a sharp picture, or if it shows too little contrast, or in any way furnishes fewer bits-per-second than it is constructed for. This apparent paradox is related to the following observation.

3. Visual information is coded in the retina before it is transmitted to the brain. In the frog, for example, single fibers of the optic nerve (between the eye and the brain) signal not just the presence of light or color in different parts of the visual image, but more complicated properties: contrast lines, moving dark objects, and other similar things [3.2]. This can be interpreted in the following way: The rods and cones of the retina deliver a surplus of information for which the repertoire of motor responses of the frog provides a poor information channel. Not everything the frog sees is relevant for the frog. To sift out what is relevant from the redundant over-production is the job of the mechanism of perception, a large part of which in the case of the frog, apparently, is contained in the retina.

Here concepts such as channel capacity, redundancy, and coding refer to an animal channel in a way that is not entirely convincing since it is disconcerting not to know who the transmitter and receiver actually are that are connected by the channel.

4. Mimicry: for example, camouflage coloring. Information about the appearance of the background on which the animal is habitually to be seen (tree bark in the case of some butterflies, etc.) is represented

on the surface of the animal to make it invisible to its natural enemies. The butterfly transfers this information genetically from generation to generation. But how did it get into the genetic text? Again: who did the transmitting? The causal analysis is complicated. It has to consider the agressors of the butterfly and their ability to discriminate forms visually, and it relies on the power of the evolutionary principles of variation and selection. This leads far from the original concept of data transmission between two people who speak the same language.

5. The brain of a species of animal is adapted to the environment in which the animal lives. The brain contains information about the structure of the environment, just as the wings of a butterfly contain pictorial information about the appearance of the bark of a tree or of a pair of frightening vertebrate animal eyes. This is particularly interesting to us brain anatomists who want to extract information from brains and even hope by this means to obtain information about the different environments in which the bearers of brains live. The brain as a model of environment, as a microcosm mirroring the macrocosm, is one of the basic themes of brain science.

But how does the information from the macrocosm get into the microcosm? Can the information about the world that a brain has received genetically, and that which it has absorbed during its life through experience, also be measured in bits? In order to progress along this line of thought I propose the following hypothetical experiment.

I imagine myself receiving information from a certain source, for example, from another human being transmitting a text to me through a teletype machine. I observe first that all the letters of our alphabet are being transmitted in an apparently haphazard succession, so many letters per second. From this, I can calculate the so-called information flow in bits per second or bit per sign times the number of the transmitted signs per second. Provided that I receive the transmitted sequence with any interest at all, this measure is a measure of the interest that the source has for me, a measure of the surprises that the source can deliver per unit of time, or in other words, a measure of my uncertainty about what is being said; which means a measure of my inability to predict what the next letter will be. After a while, I discover that the letters in the transmitted text do not by any means occur with the same frequency; that "e", for example, appears more often than "y". Then I discover that certain successions of letters occur more frequently than others, that certain letters follow certain other letters, as for example after "q" in some of our European languages, the probability that "u" will follow is very high. Every such discovery about the characteristics of the information source reduces my uncertainty in predicting the text that is being transmitted and reduces the extent of my original interest in the source. The information flow in bits per second is reduced for me, which mathematically speaking, is a consequence of the fact that if signs condition one another, certain successions of signs become more probable than others, while the maximum of (average) information per succession of signs results, according to Shannon's measure of information, if all succession of signs of a certain length are equally probable.

This process of getting acquainted with the source may continue at higher and higher levels of complexity. After a certain time I discover that it does not just transmit a succession of letters, but words of a particular language that I know (or possibly which I learn while I listen). I can now follow the text with understanding and will do that as long as I can experience surprises. The source will become ever more familiar; in the end I will be able to predict almost every word. I can then hardly learn anything new. I have no more uncertainty, I experience no surprises; the information flow of this source will, for me, tend to zero. I say, for me, because naturally someone else, who is not yet acquainted with my source, and who begins to follow it, can receive at first the full measure of information from it, as I did at the beginning.

I maintain two things: first, that the flow of information produced by a source is not a property of the source alone, but of the pair, source and receiver; second, that getting acquainted with the source destroys the flow of information.

It could be objected that I am considering a peculiar case in which rather than listening to the messages for the sake of getting information, I had the perverse intention of getting acquainted with the character of the source. I believe, however, that this aspect of getting acquainted with a partner in conversation and the consequent reduction of the information per utterance given off by the partner, is fundamental to every information process. If it is not the speaker himself, (or writer, or other producer of information) whose linguistic and other properties interest me, then it is the situation about which he informs me. This external situation can be considered as the real source of information. As long as its communication holds surprises for me, it will contain much information, but as soon as I have taken it into the memory store of my brain, it becomes predictable and, therefore, lacking in information. If, on the other hand, no part of the information gets stored, either because I am not listening, or because I do not understand, then the communication produces no effect, and one cannot speak of a transmission of information as having taken place.

This observation helps perhaps to understand in which sense information is stored in the brain and from where it comes. The process, which we have called the getting-acquainted-with-a-source-of-information, consists of the embodiment of the rules and regularities that govern the source. "To know the source" means nothing more than that one is in the position to predict, from a short utterance on the part of the source, what will be said next. Prediction means, however, that the brain of the receiver falls into a sequence of internal states of its own accord, which would otherwise be forced upon it if it continued to listen to the source. The brain of the receiver that knows the source differs from the same brain at a time before it knew the source, by a loss in freedom in the succession of states. The loss of freedom arises from the fact that the internal states of the brain, which represent the utterances of the source, are now in a causal relation to each other due to the rules incorporated in the workings of the brain. This causal relation mirrors the structure of the source. It can be said, generally, that the appearance of structure in the channel, i. e., of constraints that restrict its freedom, entails a reduction in channel capacity. Applied to the brain: the reduction of information flow from the source to the receiver, which is known as getting to know the source, goes along with a reduction of the channel capacity of the receiver's brain, i. e., with an increase in structure.

It is tempting to take the decrease of the rate of information flow as a measure of the amount of structure that has been incorporated into the brain. We cannot do this in a satisfactory way for the real brain, but we can sketch a model situation that may help clarify the concepts and that even shows how some numbers may be attached to them.[2]

We say that somebody is *informed* about a *situation* through a *message*. Let us take simple situations, simple messages, and equally simple brains. The situations are configurations of black and white squares in an array of four by four squares. As an example take the following configuration A:

FIGURE 3.1   A

---

[2]   This section is dedicated to Almut.

The messages have the same shape as the configurations, being so to speak, images of them, with numbers 0 and 1 to indicate the presence of a white or black field in the corresponding position. For example, B is a complete message about A, while C is an incomplete message since it contains empty, undefined spaces.

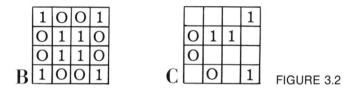

FIGURE 3.2

There are, of course, also false messages about A, but we shall not be concerned with lies or with mistakes.

We should like to say that C contains less information about A than B does. More precisely, C carries only $7/16$ of the information about A, since only seven of the 16 positions are defined, while B carries the whole information about A. If we want to call the information transmitted by the indication of the blackness or whiteness of one square "one bit", we may say that B carries 16 bits, C only 7 bits. An empty square in the message carries no information − it leaves the question completely open whether in that position the configuration is white or black: it transmits 0 bits.

Some people [3.3, 3.4] prefer to define the measure of information in terms of probabilities. The message B, they would say, specifies one particular configuration among the 2^{16} configurations that can be made by putting black and white squares in the 16 positions of the array. If we have no other knowledge, the probability that the particular configuration is the case is $1/2^{16} = 2^{-16}$. If it is agreed that the information content of a message in bits is the negative logarithm (base 2) of the probability of the situation that it specifies, one comes up again with the same result: B carries 16 bits of information.

How much information is transmitted by message C? According to our simple reasoning, 7 bits. According to the other reasoning, we have to argue thus: C leaves a lot open. C could be an incomplete message about any of the configurations that have white and black squares in the 7 positions specified by C, not just about the particular configuration A. There are 2^9 configurations about which C is a true, even if incomplete message, since C has 9 empty spaces that could be filled in so many ways with ones and zeros. The probability that a given situation should correspond to the message C is, therefore, $2^9/2^{16}$

$= 2^{-7}$ and the negative logarithm (base 2) is 7. C carries 7 bits of information, as we had already thought.

Now, it may happen that the receiver of the message already has some *knowledge* about the messages to be expected. He might know, for example, that some configurations do not occur at all. Thus we may imagine that only configurations with bilateral symmetry occur, in which case D and E are possible, F and G impossible configurations:

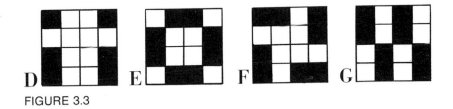

D   E   F   G

FIGURE 3.3

or only configurations in which a diagonal carries only black squares, or no black squares at all, with H as an example of a configuration that satisfies this condition, and I as one that does not.

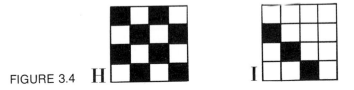

FIGURE 3.4 H   I

Bilateral symmetry reduces the possible configurations to 2^8, while the condition on the diagonals reduces the possibilities to just four configurations, the two complementary checkerboards, and the all white and all black arrays. Thus we may say that the statement that only bilaterally symmetric configurations occur in our array of 4 by 4 squares carries 8 bits of information, since it will now be necessary to specify only one-half of the squares (for instance the left half) in order to tell the whole truth about the 4 by 4 array. The statement about the diagonals being all black or all white reduces the 2^{16} configurations that are a priori possible to just 2^2 configurations: the statement is worth 14 bits. In fact, two more bits will suffice to describe the configuration that has actually occurred: a 1 and an adjacent 0 will specify one of the two checkerboard solutions, and two adjacent 1s or 0s, one of the other two solutions.

More examples: the statement that the number of black squares is odd is worth 1 bit. The indication that the configurations represent letters of the alphabet reduces the possible configuration to about 2^5 (this is largely a matter of taste) and therefore carries 11 bits. The statement that no black square has a black neighbor to its right or left carries 4 bits, as one can easily convince oneself. It is slightly more complicated to show that the condition "no black square has a black neighbor either to its right or left or above or below" leaves only 1234 possible configurations and therefore carries a little less than 6 bits.

Now we shall suppose that the receiver of the message is a simple brain consisting of 4 by 4 neurons that are activated as a consequence of the message received. All the neurons in the places corresponding to the 1s of the message become active. There will be, therefore, in the brain an image of the situation about which the message is dealing. It is clear then that we can picture the knowledge contained in the brain as a set of fibers connecting the neurons. The knowledge about bilateral symmetry, for example, could be represented by fibers

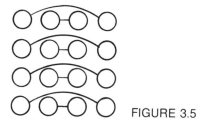

FIGURE 3.5

connecting pairs of neurons in such a way that the neuron at one end of the fiber, when it becomes active, also activates the neuron at the other end.[3] Similarly, the statement "no black square has a black neighbor" could be represented by a set of inhibitory fibers, drawn here as dotted lines that serve to inactivate all the neighbors of an active neuron.

---

[3] In real brains, each of these lines would have to be represented by two fibers, one for each direction.

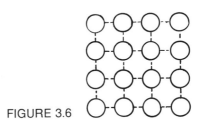

FIGURE 3.6

It is clear from these examples how the reduction of the freedom of the brain that is obtained by coupling the neurons through fibers may be compared to the reduction of freedom of the source, which goes by the name of redundancy. In the first example, each of the fibers connecting pairs of neurons has incorporated one bit into the brain, in the second case, each inhibitory connection is worth, on the average, a little less than $1/4$ of a bit.

References

3.1 Anaxagoras, In: Nahm, M. C. Selections from Early Greek Philosophy. 4th ed., New York: Meredith Publ. Comp., 1964, p. 134

3.2 Lettvin, J. Y., Maturana, H. R., McCulloch, W. S., Pitts, W. H.: What the frog's eye tells the frog's brain. Proc. Inst. Rad. Engrs. *47*, 1940–1951 (1959)

3.3 Shannon, C. E., Weaver, W.: The Mathematical Theory of Communication, Urbana: Univ. Illinois Press 1949

3.4 Wiener, N.: Cybernetics. New York-London: M. I. T. Press and Wiley 1948 (1961)

4. What Brains Are Made Of

*The fine structure of the grey substance of the brain
is not the same all over. Basically, it consists of nerve
fibers . . . of strange granula, of ganglion cells, and
of an apparently homogenous, structureless molecular mass, an unusually fine network, in which the
finest terminations of the white nerve fibers and the
ramifications of the ganglion-cell processes dis-
solve.* Griesinger, 1861 [4.3]

*. . . Most likely these millions of cells are connected
with one another.* Krafft-Ebing, 1897 [4.6]

*The more one finds out about properties of different
synapses, the less grows one's inclination to make
general statements about their mode of action.*
Katz, 1966 [4.5]

All brains are surprisingly similar. Once one has seen histologic
preparations of human brain under the microscope, one will have no
trouble recognizing nerve tissue of other animals even in species that
are only very distantly related to us, such as squids or insects. I shall
try to give a general characterization of nerve tissue.

The striking thing about brains is their fibrous structure. Brains
consist almost exclusively of fibers. The human brain for example is
made of about a million kilometers of fibers, as is easily calculated if
one takes a thousandth of a millimeter as the average thickness of the
fibers, and 1.3 liters as the volume of the brain. The fibers of a single
human brain placed end to end would form a string that could be
looped from the earth around the moon and back. The sum of the
lengths of the fibers of all living human brains, 100 light years, could
span the distance between us and neighboring stars of our galaxy.

There are other organs with a fibrous texture such as muscles or
tendons. Their function is known to be mechanical and has something
to do with forces that act in the longitudinal direction of the fiber. For
this reason muscle or tendon fibers tend to be arranged in parallel
bundles, and the fibers work together in a very simple way. The luxu-

riant branching that characterizes nerve fibers is missing in muscle and connective tissue. The fiber felt that results from this ramification gives the nerve tissue its particular character.

There are two kinds of fibrous branched cells in the nerve tissue: the glia cells and the nerve cells or neurons. Although the number of glia cells exceeds that of neurons, there will be hardly any mention of them in the rest of this book. In different regions in the brains of different vertebrates a relation of glia cells to nerve cells was found that varied between $1:1$ and $40:1$.[4] It is not surprising that every so often someone attempts to revolutionize our ideas about the brain by ascribing to the glia the essential secrets of brain function. One knows so little about these small companions to the neurons that the most diverse theories are possible and at present cannot be disproved. One should, however, keep in mind the fact that glia cells increase greatly in number whenever the nerve tissue becomes functionless due to a lesion or an interruption of the blood supply that has caused many neurons to die. In such cases the glia replaces the neurons, but certainly does not take over their function. In healthy tissue, physiologists studying electric phenomena in glia cells could not find any indication that the glia had any other part in the complex interplay of electric signals in neurons than that of foraging for the neurons. What is certain is that the glia cells envelop the nerve fibers, separate neighboring neurons from each other, and construct an insulating sheath around many nerve fibers made of layers of a fatty substance called myelin.

The main reason why we do not want to occupy ourselves further with the glia cells is their great uniformity compared to the variety of shapes of the neurons. The small star-shaped glia cells are scattered among the neurons more or less in the same manner throughout the nervous system; if one were to look only at them, forgetting the nerve cells, a much more uniform description of the different parts of the nervous system would be obtained than one based on a description of the neurons. If the aim is to relate different structures to different tasks, one is certainly better off concentrating on the neurons.

The fibrous structure of brains is related to a functional principle that could be called the principle of addressed communication. This is a characteristic that brains have in common with digital computers. Signals are transmitted from every point of the brain to one or more definite other points. Messages "to whom it may concern", typical for

---

[4]   cf. Reference [4.1]. Those who miss tables and graphs in the present essay are urged to consult this very useful book.

the hormonal system, or for the signal transmission through odors in the sex life of many animals certainly play a lesser role in the brain. The image of a cosmic cloud made of matter with a diffuse structure but endowed with a complex internal radio communications system enabling it to think, appears in a novel by an astronomer, but does not convince the brain anatomist. One has the feeling that the high specificity of point-to-point connections available in a structure made of wires or fibers could hardly be matched by the specific resonance of transmitters and receivers tuned to a set of radio frequencies.

If the transmission of messages inside the brain takes place not in a three-dimensional continuum, but in a system of isolated wires, the question may still be asked, whether or not these wires are connected end to end in such a way as to make a net without interruptions. Speaking of nerve cells: do they form a syncytium in which the cell boundaries are abolished, or do they maintain their individuality in the nerve net? The latter is true, as had long been supposed, but certainty was provided only by the electron microscope. At the high magnification afforded by electron microscopy it can clearly be seen that where two nerve cells touch, the cell membranes may lie close together, but they are never fused into one common membrane with an opening that would allow a free exchange of cellular material [4.7]. In fact, they are frequently insulated from each other by a flattened piece of glia cell.

This finding leads to a general statement about the function of nerve fibers. It is to be expected that signals running along one nerve fiber are carried by a different mechanism from that which relays the signals from one neuron to the next.

From the vast body of facts collected by the electrophysiologists I will try to make an extract that will show that actually not less than 5 different kinds of signal transmission can be distinguished within the nervous system.[5]

First a few introductory remarks about the actual signal carrier, the membrane of the nerve cell are in order. As with other cell types, this thin skin, consisting of several layers of different molecules and sheathing the entire neuron, controls the transport of substances into and out of the cell. Thus, the cell membrane plays a crucial role by guarding the frontier between the organism and its environment. The proteins in the membrane certainly play an important part in this,

---

[5] For those who desire more detailed information, I highly recommend Reference [4.5].

both in the case when the membrane acts as a passive filter that sets up a greater or lesser resistance to the passage of different kinds of particles, and in the case in which the membrane interferes actively in the transport, i. e., when the energy for the movement of the particle comes from the membrane itself. What interests us particularly is the role of the cell membrane in the generation of the electric potential that can be found in all cells. The interior of the cell is normally negative with respect to the outside. This potential collapses as soon as the cell dies, and is apparently due to an active separation of ions by the membrane. It is certain that the membrane potential has something to do with the fact that Na^+ ions have a higher concentration outside the cell and K^+ ions inside. Starting from a condition in which both ions inside and outside the cell are equally concentrated, the active interference of the cell membrane soon shifts the balance. A simple explanation of how this comes about is that of a sodium pump in the membrane, which continuously transports Na^+ ions from inside to outside, and thus charges the membrane positively. The K^+ ions, according to this theory, passively follow the electrostatic force produced by this charge and pile up inside the cell. Another hypothesis is that of a sodium-potassium pump in the membrane that continously discharges Na^+ ions from the cell while it brings in an equal quantity of K^+ ions. According to this theory, the symmetric movement of two positive ions indirectly generates the charge of the membrane, which results from the different mobilities of Na^+ and K^+ ions through the membrane. The potassium ions pumped into the cell permeate out much faster than the sodium ions permeate in. This causes a steady surplus of positive ions as long as the sodium-potassium pump is in action and as long as nothing happens to change the membrane's differential permeability for the two kinds of ions. Since a relatively superficial knowledge of the physiology of the neuronal membrane suffices for our purposes, it is not necessary to make a choice for one or the other theory of origin of the membrane potential (in fact, several alternative theories have been proposed lately). It is sufficient to know that the different kinds of signals that we assume to be the main carriers of information within the nervous system are essentially perturbations of the membrane potential (the so-called resting potential) of the nerve cells. Signal transmission takes place on the surface of the neurons. We are less well informed about the role of the processes inside the neurons, which occur at a slower pace than those in the membrane. It is likely that these processes are involved with growth and nourishment of the neurons, rather than with the quick workings of information processing in the brain.

The first and most impressive disturbance of the resting potential of the neuronal cell membrane is called *action potential* in textbooks and "spike" in laboratory jargon. The term spike refers to the shape of the peaks that are seen on the oscillograph records when the membrane potential is measured by a fine electrode placed in the vicinity, or in the interior of the neuron. (The more interpretable records of the membrane potential are obtained by means of one electrode inside the cell and one outside, which may be placed at some distance and is then called "indifferent electrode".) This peak is generated by the rapid decay of the membrane potential, followed by a reversal of the potential for a short time, and by its return to the previous polarity within about a thousandth of a second. The phenomenon is not completely over in a millisecond, as witnessed by the slow oscillations of the membrane potential that follow each spike. These so-called after-potentials last about 100 ms and accompany the restoration of the status quo after the catastrophic event of the spike.

Spikes can appear either singly or in rapid succession, up to several hundred per second. When they occur in such rapid sequences, the spikes step on each other's tails, so to speak, since the oscillation of one is not finished before the next one starts. This situation can be sustained only over a short period. Under normal circumstances of activation many neurons tend to generate 10 spikes or less per second so that each spike is able to complete its entire cycle without interference from the following one.

All the spikes of a sequence produced by one and the same neuron look almost identical. They change their shape only in exceptional circumstances, e. g., at very high spike frequencies. Spikes are also similar in different neurons, although there are certain types of neurons in which the whole process occurs more slowly than in others.

What is the nature of this explosive phenomenon that so radically changes the membrane potential? A great deal of biophysics has been lavished upon this problem, and information about it can be gained from References [4.4] and [4.5]. The spike is set off by an increase of the permeability for sodium ions in the membrane. The lock that has prevented the entrance of positive sodium ions through the resting membrane to the negative interior of the cell, suddenly opens. Na^+ streams inward, the surplus of positive ions outside decreases rapidly, and briefly, a surplus is created inside. Very soon, however, something happens that works against this current of positive charges: shortly after the sodium lock opens, the potassium lock also opens far wider than in a state of rest. K^+ diffuses outward and the membrane turns positive again on the outside. These dramatic events are followed by the slower process of again tidying and sorting the ionic species, by which the original imbalance of ions inside and outside the membrane is reestablished. The explosive dynamics of the spike is due to a positive feedback: what has already been produced is the cause of more of the same being produced. The permeability of the membrane for sodium ions depends strongly on the membrane potential, in the sense that it increases as the potential difference between inside and outside decreases. On the other hand, the membrane potential itself changes with the influx of positive sodium ions into the cell. The potential decreases, causing a further opening of the sodium lock etc. The vicious circle builds up to the catastrophic event that is recorded as a spike on the oscillograph. The positive feedback remains in action until it is interrupted by a negative one; the opening of the potassium lock has this function since it starts the flow of positive ions from the inside out, and thus brings the membrane potential back to its original charge in the short time of a millisecond.

It is easy to understand how a spike can be generated in a neuron by the most diverse stimuli. All that is needed is to raise the permeability of the membrane for sodium ions by chemical or mechanical means and everything else happens accordingly. The membrane potential can be changed by applying an electric field that works against the resting potential. As soon as a critical threshold of the membrane potential is undercut, the change in the permeability for sodium is large enough to start off the catastrophic cycle.

Up to now we have seen how spikes arise locally on the nerve cell membrane, but not how they travel along the nerve fiber. This they do, acting as signals in the central and peripheral nervous system. It seems that the currents of ions across the membrane that accompany the spike cause a disturbance of the membrane potential in the surrounding area of membrane not directly involved in the spike. There, in turn, another spike is produced. Actually, the spike runs as a wave over the whole fiber and appears at different places exactly in the same form, only delayed. Intensity is not lost on the way, since the spike's energy is drawn from the electrical charge of the membrane and is continuously regenerated on the way. In most cases the spike-wave runs into all branches of a nerve fiber with undiminished amplitude. In this way, signals can be duplicated without the copies having to share the energy of their parent signal. This property of nerve fibers must fill communication engineers with envy. If lines of this sort were available to them, they could construct networks according to the demands of the logical design without ever having to bother with the problem of how to keep up with the energy supply.

A fiber conducting a spike acts more like a fuse than like an electric conductor. A fuse transmits the "signal", i.e., the fire with undiminished strength into all of its ramifications. The comparison with a fuse also makes it clear what price has to be paid for signal transmission untroubled by problems of energy. When the wick has burned out it has to be replaced. This takes time. Analogously, the processes that replenish the energy in the nerve fiber after each spike, in order to make it ready for the next spike, set an upper limit to the information a nerve fiber can transmit within a certain time.

A second mode of signal transmission in a neuron is *electrotonic transmission,* or *conduction with decrement.* Under certain circumstances, no spike is generated by the depolarization of the membrane. This may depend on different characteristics of the membrane in different parts of the neuron, or just on the strength of the excitation. In fact, when the depolarization does not reach a certain threshold value, a local disturbance is produced that is not transmitted as a spike, but decreases in intensity with the distance from the point of stimulation (decrement = decrease). Such a wave of depolarization decays in a few milliseconds, whereby the time course also changes with the distance from the origin: it becomes slower the further away it is recorded. The whole phenomenon can be easily understood if one thinks of the membrane as consisting only of resistances and capacitors, and if one forgets the power supply built into the membrane, which we have seen in operation during the spike-discharge.

The third manner of signal transmission is from neuron to neuron through *electric synapses.* Synapse means somewhat ambiguously, both the functional connection between neurons, and the site where the action of one neuron upon another takes place. The transmission of the disturbance of the membrane potential from one cell to its neighbor in the case of electric synapses can be explained by the transmitting mechanism already described. This applies to the spike as well as to the lower-than-threshold electrotonic transmission. Direct electric coupling naturally occurs whenever the individual cells have grown together to form a *syncytium,* that is, when their membranes have fused into a continuous, common membrane as is the case with giant nerve fibers originally built up from several cells. The condition for direct transmission by currents of ions is much less favorable if two nerve fibers are in close contact without actually having a direct cytoplasmic connection. Even so, there is the possibility of electric coupling if the fibers are large in diameter and/or the space that separates them is very small. In fact, in cases where direct electric transmission has been demonstrated, points have been found by high resolution

electron microscopy on the surface of the cell where the membranes
of neighboring neurons appear to be stuck.

In some cases of so-called electric synapses, conditions are further
complicated by the fact that the electric connection does not have the
same transmission characteristics in both directions, although this
asymmetry is not evident in the microscopic picture of the synapse.
The following conclusion of Katz applies particularly to the electric
synapses: "the more one learns about the characteristics of different
synapses, the less one is prone to make general statements about their
manner of functioning."

The fourth type of signal transmission is from neuron to neuron by
means of *excitatory chemical synapses.* Synapses in which transmitter
substance is released that acts as a messenger between one neuron
and the next are certainly more important in the central nervous system than the synapses with purely electric coupling. Chemical transmission was first described in a particular sort of synapse at the margin of the nervous system: in the transmission from nerve to muscle.
Acetylcholine was recognized as the substance released at the nerve
endings when the nerve was stimulated. It reaches the cell membrane
of the muscle and sets the process in motion that results in the con-
traction of the muscle. Although the idea that certain chemicals
(transmitter substances, as they are often called) are also used in signal transmission from neuron to neuron within the nervous system has
been useful in interpreting many electrophysiologic and microscopic
findings, the actual transmitter in most instances has, as yet, not been
identified. The best-known synapses are those of the motoneurons of
the spinal cord. The cell bodies of these neurons are large and may be
easily penetrated by small electric probes (microelectrodes). Thus,
when the fibers that are connected synaptically with the motoneurons
are stimulated, the changes of the membrane potential can be observed within the target neurons, i. e., beyond the synapse. The transmission of excitation from neuron to neuron is best explained by the following chain of events: a spike in a fiber leading to the motoneuron
induces the terminal part of this fiber to release a small amount of
a transmitter substance. This changes the characteristics of the membrane of the motoneuron at the point of contact by increasing its permeability for sodium ions. If the action of the transmitter substance
was strong enough (e. g., if a large enough number of afferent fibers
were simultaneously activated), the membrane potential of the motoneuron will be lowered enough in one point to produce a spike which
then spreads into the axon. The transmitter substance disappears within a few milliseconds, being probably broken up by enzymes as in the

case of acetylcholine in the neuromuscular synapse. More information about the motoneuron of the cat and its synapses can be found in Reference [4.2].

The fifth type of signal transmission is *inhibition* by means of chemical synapses. This, too, is well known from investigations on the motoneuron of the cat. A part of the fibers leading to the motoneuron influence it negatively in the sense that the stimulation of these fibers makes it less likely or even impossible for a spike to arise in the motoneuron. This is certainly due to a transmitter substance that changes something in the permeability of the membrane for ions. Thus, there are at least two (and most probably a few more) different transmitters in the central nervous system: one that excites, and one that inhibits the target neuron. Whether each transmitter is produced by a special category of neurons or whether the same neuron can generate excitation and inhibition in different synaptic contacts is as yet unknown.

Following our initial intention of learning to read the meaning of the brain from its structure, we may now ask the next question: is there a dictionary that allows us to translate different forms of fibers as seen in histologic preparations and different appearances of the synaptic apparatuses into the different kinds of signal transmissions described above? Can one tell by looking at a fiber if it is capable of generating spikes, or if it only conveys electrotonic variations in the membrane potential? Can the point of contact between two neurons reveal whether or not a synapse occurs there, and what type of synapse?

The kind of answer one obtains depends very much on whom one asks. A neuroanatomist who thinks only in terms of vertebrate brains would tend to be confident that he can tell the difference between nerve cell processes that conduct spikes and those that conduct electrotonically, and in most cases he will also be able to determine the direction of conduction from the histologic picture. If we ask someone who works with insect or other invertebrate brains, we will receive a much more tentative answer. We shall stick to the experience on vertebrate brains, since a great deal of research has already been concentrated on the nervous systems of man, cat, and frog. It is perhaps more feasible at present to make correlations between anatomy and neurophysiology in vertebrates than in crabs, insects, or octopuses.

Digression on Techniques in the Histology of the Nervous System. Looking at the consistency of a brain at the butcher's we do not get the idea that there is an enormous amount of structure to be discovered there. How may we discover the wealth of fibrous connections in this soft mass, which for centuries was supposed.to be nothing but slime to cool the hot vapors of the heart? Here is a summary of the most important procedures that have been developed over the last hundred years for studying brain structure. Common to all of them is the *fixation* of the tissue immediately after death, a process involving the denaturation of proteins and polymerization of various tissue components with the aim of creating an irreversible condition, at the same time preserving as much as possible of the original structure. For this, alcohol may be used, or mixtures of alcohol, acetic acid, and chloroform, or potassium dichromate (a substance traditionally used for tanning), and especially the aldehydes: formaldehyde and, recently, glutaraldehyde, which are best injected into the tissue through the circulatory system. This procedure is also called "hardening" since the nerve tissue after fixation acquires a greater consistency. It is still, however, too soft for cutting and must therefore be embedded in liquid paraffin, celloidin, or synthetic resin. The solidified block is then cut with the aid of a microtome in series of sections whose thickness varies, according to the method used, from 0.05–100 µm.

Staining Techniques. Nerve tissue is everywhere transparent to visible light as well as to electrons. In other words, not much would be seen in the light- or electron microscope unless certain components of the tissue were stained beforehand with a light-absorbing or electron-scattering substance. Preparation of nerve tissue for the electron microscope involves mainly staining of cell membranes by means of heavy-metal ions. In light microscopy stains are used that have specific affinities for various cell types or parts of cells. The *Nissl procedure* stains certain components of the cell nucleus, making it possible to count neurons. Other stains are specific for *myelin*, the insulating material that encases many nerve fibers. Various procedures using silver salts have been especially useful in the analysis of nerve nets. They

▶

FIGURE 4.1. A typical vertebrate neuron, consisting of a dendritic tree (*d*), a cell body (*s*) containing the nucleus, axon (*a*) with a branch or axon collateral (*c*) and with terminal arborizations (*t*). The myelin sheath of the axon is interrupted in several places (*n*), among other also at the branching point. The single parts of the neuron are drawn in realistic proportions to each other: the dendritic tree has a diameter of about 400 µm, the axon is 10 mm long (cut up in 20 pieces of 0.5 mm each) and the two terminal arborizations have a diameter of 200 µm each. The thickness of the axon, without the myelin sheath, is 1 µm

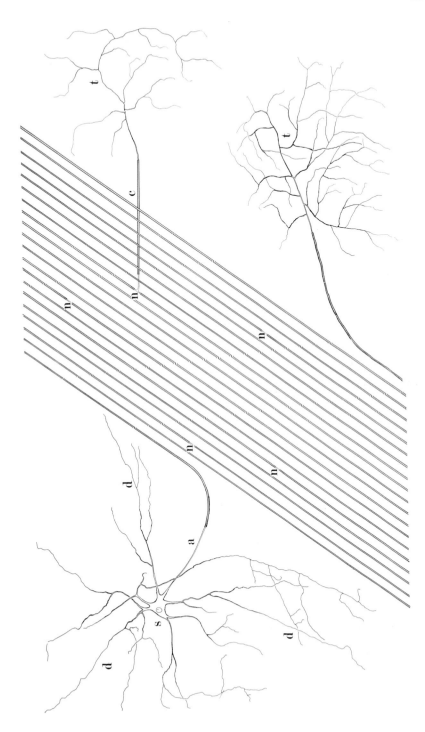

are based not so much on a chemical affinity as on the tendency of silver to percipitate along thread-like or tubular formations such as nerve fibers (also glia and connective tissue fibers, etc.).

The *Golgi method* deserves special mention since it alone has probably yielded as much information about the fine structure of the brain as all the other methods taken together. It isolates single neurons from the tangled net arising from the close interweaving of many star-shaped elements (the neurons) by filling some with a reddish black precipitate and leaving the remaining tissue completely unstained. This peculiar behavior of the Golgi stain is probably due to the accidental formation of nuclei of precipitation in various places in the tissue, and to the fact that the further extension of the precipitate (silver chromate) remains confined by the cell membrane once it has started inside a cell. If we have many preparations, each showing single representatives of different kinds of neurons, a complete picture of the tangled net in the nerve tissue can be reconstructed.

Finally, methods have been used that take advantage of the particular stainability of injured or dead neurons (so-called degeneration methods). A lesion is made in a certain place in the brain of a living animal. After days or weeks, depending on the method used, the animal is sacrificed, and the brain is searched for degenerated neurons. A picture can thus be obtained of the fiber connections between the place of the lesion and other parts of the brain, since only these show up in the sections after the specific staining method has been applied.

Other methods have recently been developed for much the same purpose that take advantage of the active uptake and transport within the neuron of certain substances that are applied locally in the brain. Certain amino acids, applied in the vicinity of the cell body, travel within the neuron into all the ramifications of the axon, while an enzyme, horseradish peroxydase, can be used to follow fibers in the opposite direction, since it is taken up by the axonal terminations and conveyed toward the nucleus.

▶

FIGURE 4.2. Two neurons from the cortex of a female *Bos taurus* (cow) in a Golgi preparation. The larger neuron, to the right, is a pyramidal cell with a descending axon (*a*) and an axon collateral (*c*). A dendrite of the same neuron (*d*) is covered with spines, most of the other dendrites are out of focus. The smaller neuron to the left has a spindle-shaped cell body (*s*) and thinner dendrites. Its axon is not within the focal plane. The optical resolution of the micrograph is not very satisfactory, since to obtain the necessary depth of focus for fibers that are not quite parallel to the imaging plane, the aperture of the lens has to be reduced

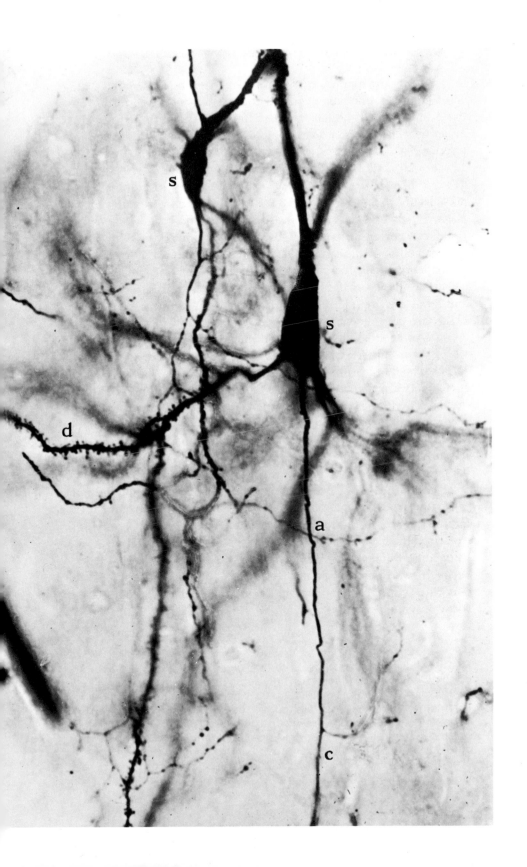

I would now like to describe a typical neuron (Figs. 4.1, 4.2) that will summarize the main characteristics of most neurons of the vertebrate brain. Even though this description does not apply directly to insect neurons, it can at least be used as the foundation for a common terminology.

The cell body (s) is the only thickening of the otherwise very slender tree-like structure of a neuron. In vertebrates it encloses the cell nucleus. Its size varies from 5 to 100 μm in diameter. Neurons with larger ramifications usually have larger cell bodies; the same applies to the cell nucleus.

The cell body has several extensions. One, the axon (a), is distinguished from the others by its length (it is often very much longer), sometimes by its smaller caliber, often by the pattern of its branching, and always by the fact that the thickness of every piece between one branching point and the next remains constant. Thus the axonal tree consists of cylindrical segments, with the exception of the initial part, which is conical. The number of its branches varies with different neuron types between very few and several hundred; the length (maximal extension from the cell body) may vary between 0.1 mm and several meters. The branches of the axon may all be concentrated in a narrow region, or may be distributed very loosely over a large space. The branching is always tree-like, not net-like: the terminations of different branches of the same neuron never fuse, so that closed circuits within the same neuron never arise.

The other cell processes that can arise singly or severally from the cell body are called *dendrites* (d). The most dependable characteristic that makes it possible to distinguish even small parts of the dendritic tree from axonal ramifications, is the tendency of dendritic branches to become thinner with increasing distance from the cell body, also between two branching points. There are, however, exceptions: long dendritic segments that maintain a constant caliber (e. g., the shaft of cortical pyramidal cells, see Chapt. 8). Another distinguishing characteristic of dendrites, which is not, however, true of all neuron types,

▶

FIGURE 4.3. Two dendrites from a Golgi preparation of the mouse cortex. The Golgi method stains only some of the neurons present in the tissue in an apparently unsystematic way. If one imagines the whole volume densely packed with dendrites, crossing each other in all directions, and if one adds to this picture an equal amount of axonal fibers interwoven with the dendritic felt, one obtains a realistic picture of the cortical neuropil. The two dendrites have different thickness, but are both densely covered with spines. There are about two spines on every μm of dendritic length

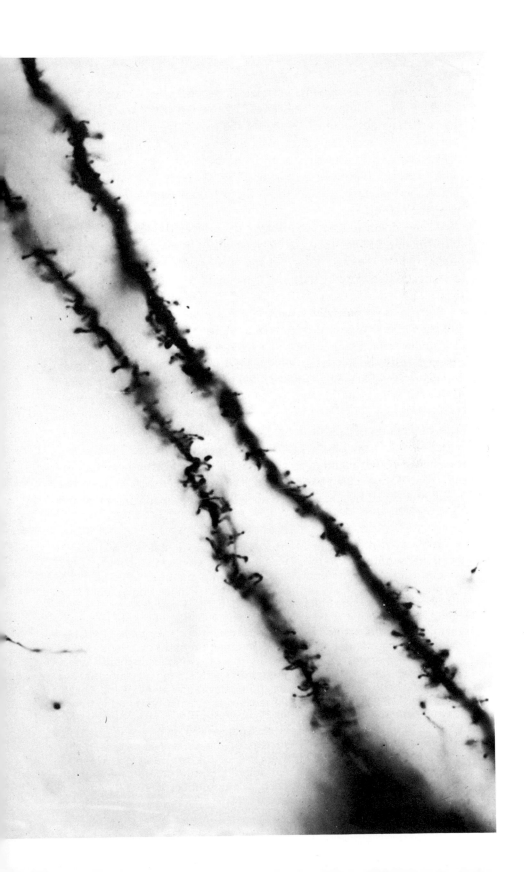

are the so-called spines (Fig. 4.3), which decorate the surface of dendrites in great numbers. The length of the dendritic processes also varies, though not so much as that of the axons, from about 10 μm to several millimeters. Dendritic trees also take many different forms: radially symmetric dendrites distributed around the cell body, or two main branches placed at opposite sides of the cell body, or a rich ramification at some distance from the cell body connected to it only by a single trunk, etc.

Axons, dendrites, and cell bodies are sufficiently different in their fine structure so that they can be recognized in electron microscopic pictures where the macroscopic shape of the neuron is no help in their identification because of the excessive magnification and small field of view.

We can now partially answer the question as to whether, from looking at the anatomical picture of a neuron, we can infer what kind of stimulus transmission occurs at a given point. A large body of experimental facts supports the opinion held by most neurophysiologists that axons conduct spikes, whereas dendrites are not normally capable of this. As a rule, in vertebrates the dendrites of one neuron receive signals from other neurons and conduct these to the cell body in the form of graded changes of the membrane potential. There the signals come together from all the branches of the dendritic tree. In this way, the change of the membrane potential also reaches the beginning of the axon, the so-called axon hillock, where it releases a spike if the intensity reaches the threshold. The spike then spreads undiminished

▶

FIGURE 4.4. Two synapses in the second visual ganglion, the medulla ganglionaris, of the fly. In the places marked s, a presynaptic and a postsynaptic neuron are in direct apposition, not separated by the lamellae of other cells, l, which are probably mostly glia. Proceeding in the direction of the arrows, the following components of the synapse are encountered: an axonal region (a) containing synaptic vesicles (v), a presynaptic structure, stained rather darkly, which has the shape of a table (inverted in the picture) standing on the membrane on two legs (lower synapse) or one leg (upper synapse), the presynaptic membrane, the synaptic cleft, the postsynaptic membrane with some fuzzy material attached to it, and the cytoplasm of the postsynaptic element (d). These are probably chemical synapses. The vesicles (v) may contain the transmitter substance that is probably released into the postsynaptic cleft at the site of the synapse. In the lower synapse one gains the impression that the vesicle between the two legs of the table was caught in the process of doing just that. The shapes of the pre- and postsynaptic structures are variable in different animals and in different regions of the nervous system. m: mitochondria; t: microtubuli. × 70,000 (electron micrograph by Dr. J. Campos-Ortega)

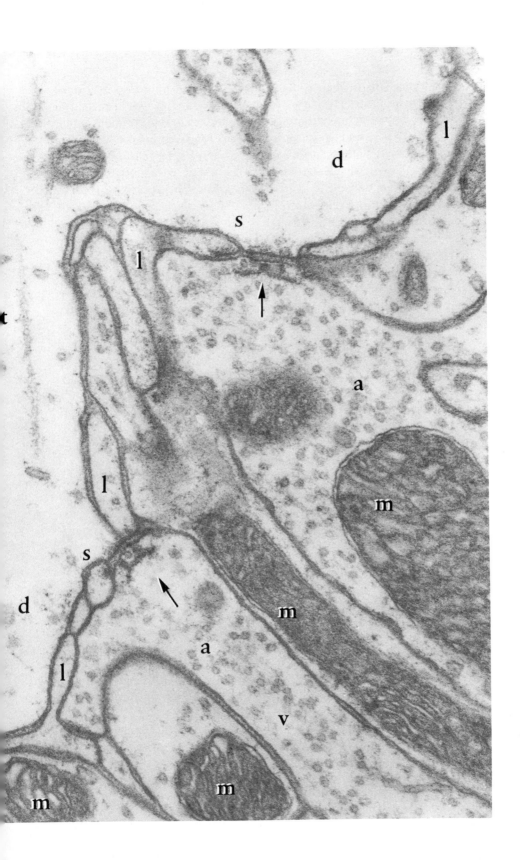

to all extensions of the axonal branching of that neuron. Because of this predetermined direction of signal transmission within a neuron from the dendritic branches to the axon and on to the axonal termination, it is to be expected that the transmission from neuron to neuron occurs through synapses in which the axonal branches of one neuron relay the signals to the dendrites of another. In fact, synapses are found at the axodendritic contact points, frequently on the surface of the spines when present, which would explain these peculiar dendritic appendages. The synapses (Figs. 4.4 and 8.4) are clearly asymmetric, i. e., different structures can be observed on the side of the axon and on that of the dendrite where the "synaptic" contact takes place. These structural specializations at the site of the synapse are useful in recognizing synapses in the electron microscope, but as yet no convincing explanation of their function has been found. They may take the shape of a dense layer of an unknown substance lining the dendritic membrane, or of a symmetric thickening of both the axonal and the dendritic membranes, or of plates of an equally unknown substance situated within the axon at a certain distance from the membrane. Only the so-called synaptic vesicles that are contained in clusters within the axon in the vicinity of the synaptic sites, may receive a fairly plausible explanation. They are characteristic for chemical synapses and probably contain synaptic transmitter substance. Occasionally such a vesicle is seen to release its contents in the synaptic cleft between the membrane of the axon and that of the dendrite: evidence perhaps of a last signal transmission at the moment of death. The explanation of the synaptic vesicles as packages of transmitter substance is made plausible by the findings at the neuromuscular synapses. There, too, vesicles can occasionally be found emptying their contents into the synaptic cleft. Also, the effect on the muscle has been shown to be produced in small doses, the amount of which is compatible with the idea that each corresponds to the bursting of one vesicle filled with acetylcholine [4.5].

This brings us further along in our quest for an anatomical–physiologic dictionary. Chemical synapses can be recognized, and the direction of signal transmission can also be determined by histologic analysis. Unfortunately, excitatory synapses can still not be distinguished reliably from inhibitory ones, either by the size of the vesicles, as was repeatedly suggested, or by the shape of the membrane thickenings. This is the most deplorable gap in the histophysiologic dictionary.

Electric synapses, on the other hand, can probably be recognized by the particularly narrow synaptic cleft.

An additional entry can be made in the histophysiologic dictionary regarding the relation of the axon to spike transmission. The form of a certain type of neuronal cell process tells us not only that it is an axon and that it may therefore generate spikes, but also something about the speed of conduction. Other things being equal, conduction is faster the thicker the fiber. A linear, or a quadratic dependance of the velocity of conduction on the diameter of the fiber has been proposed by different authors. Furthermore many fibers are encased for certain parts of their length in a sleeve of insulating material, the so-called myelin sheath (Fig. 4.1). The effect of this is that the explosive process of the spike generation jumps from one interruption of the insulation (the so-called node of Ranvier) to the next, with a consequent increase in the speed of conduction. In myelinated fibers, too, the speed increases with the increase in the diameter of the fiber. The whole range of velocities of conduction goes from less than one meter per second in thin, naked fibers to over a hundred meters per second in the thickest myelinated fibers.

These relatively safe identifications of histologic details with specialized functions relate to the nervous systems of vertebrates. The situation is less clear with invertebrates. The cell nucleus of most invertebrate neurons lies in a special sack far removed from the ramification of the neuron and connected to it by merely a thin fiber. This makes the cell body less definable so that it cannot be used as in vertebrates as a fixed point from which to find one's bearings. The differences in external form and fine structure between dendrites and axons, as we have described them for the vertebrate neuron, cannot be carried over to invertebrates, and perhaps the clear functional polarization of the neuron is indeed an advance made by vertebrates. Synapses are, however, surprisingly similar in all animals.

Gray and White Matter. A cursory glance at vertebrate brains immediately reveals two kinds of brain substances, easily distinguished even on unstained cuts. One substance appears whitish-yellow, the other appears pinkish in fresh brains. Only after the brain has been fixed in formaldehyde do the terms gray and white matter have their justification. The relative proportions of gray and white matter are about equal. The difference between the two substances becomes more obvious on microscopic examination. The gray matter contains all neural cell bodies, all dendrites, and all axonal terminations. This means that all synapses are also found here. The white matter consists only of fibers, mainly unbranched fibers surrounded mostly by a sheath of myelin. There is no evidence of reciprocal influence of the activity of neighboring fibers in the white matter, although the possibility of electrical interference of signals traveling in fibers running parallel to each other has frequently been considered. The distinction between white and gray matter is tantamount to a spatial separation of two processes: (1) the projection of signal patterns without interaction of parts of the pattern and (2) computation (or "nervous integration" as this has been often called in neurology). A similar separation can also be observed in insect brains where even three kinds of substances can be distinguished: a kind of gray matter, the so-called neuropil or fiber felt in which synapses are found (but no cell bodies), a kind of white substance (however without myelin), which serves merely to map different neuropils onto each other (e. g., the chiasmata in the visual system of the fly) and a *third substance*, which contains the nerve cell nuclei in apparently random heaps. Each nucleus is contained in a small cytoplasmic sack that sends out a slender fiber to the corresponding dendritic and axonal neuronal tree in the neuropil.

There is a common characteristic of gray matter that is independent of the particular patterns of connectivity in different regions and in different animals. The cytoplasmic processes (axons and dendrites) of the neurons in the gray matter are much longer than the average distance of the neurons from each other. This fact determines the close weave of the fiber felt in the gray matter that makes structural analysis so difficult, and that is certainly related to the very nature of the computation in the brain.

The transmission and transformation of information in a piece of gray matter certainly happens in a different way from that in the large bundles of fibers in the white matter. Neurons in one region of gray matter depend more closely on each other than on neurons in other regions. Here we become aware of the lack of terminology that would allow us to define different patterns of connectivity and to distinguish different modes of interaction other than with vague terms such as "more or less closely." Theorists have sometimes been drawn toward attempting a clarification of concepts in this field, but so far their conceptual constructs have hardly been taken over by brain scientists.

It is to be expected that shape and functional properties of single neurons will only be fully understood once an explanation in terms of the cooperative activity of the entire neuronal network can be formulated. It may well be that the function of individual neurons considered in isolation is sufficiently well described by the few cursory remarks that I have given and that the main surprises that physiology has in store for us will be in the field of many-neuron interaction rather than in that of single-neuron physiology.

I would like to conclude this Chapter with a summary sketch of the neuron such as the neuroanatomist should have in mind when attempting functional explanations of brain structures.

The neuron receives a cloud of individual signals via its dendritic tree from a very large area compared with the distance between the neuron and its neighbors. These signals are conducted with decrement, i. e., with diminishing intensity to the root of the dendritic tree, where they are all added together. The exact distribution of signals on the many synapses (up to 10^5) of the dendritic tree is lost in the process, since many different patterns of excitation yield the same value after summation at the root of the dendritic tree.

The activation of a few synapses near the root of the dendritic tree is equivalent to the activation of many synapses in distant branches, the latter being less effective because of decremental conduction. Thus, the dendritic tree plays an interesting double role: on the one hand, it is a detector of precisely localized point-like signals; on the other, it is a feeler for diffuse clouds of signals that range around the same point. One is reminded of the interplay between vague feelings and precise knowledge that we can observe in our own thinking.

The result of the computation by the dendritic tree of the distribution of excitation in the neighborhood of the neuron is conducted further to the initial segment of the axon, the critical part of the neuron. Here a spike is generated if the excitation surpasses a certain threshold, and if the same neuron has not already given off a spike shortly before. The mechanism for producing spikes is affected by a period of refractoriness that we have not yet mentioned. A continuously varying level of excitation is converted into a series of spikes separated by intervals that reflect the refractory state of the axon following each spike. The higher the average excitation level, the shorter the intervals between successive spikes. This means that information about the level of excitation of the neuron is contained as frequency modulation in the spike series generated by the neuron. Is this then the form in which a typical neuron communicates information? Yes and no. In the periphery, in the sense organs, one can generally observe how different intensities of a certain sensory quality are coded in different spike frequencies. These frequencies typically range around 10 per s. Since the spike series are also fairly irregular, several seconds are necessary before the intensity is defined with adequate precision by the average frequency of the spike series. Neurons are slow as frequency modulation channels. If one takes the sum of the spike frequencies of several parallel nerve fibers, the frequency modulation functions somewhat better, but this game cannot be carried very far since by coupling neurons together, the system loses in spatial resolution what it gains in the frequency domain. Evidently, quick perceptions and rapid decisions are mediated by a mechanism that is not based on frequency modulation. In many situations single spikes can probably trigger a reaction. Psychologists find reaction times of the order of 0.1 s between the reception of a complex signal in a sensory system and the motor response to it. This corresponds to the time between two successive spikes in a neuron firing at a moderate level of excitation. Apparently, the relevant information to which the subject reacts in a reaction-time experiment is carried by the first spike, or more likely, by the first spikes in several parallel channels.

Here we find again, in the time domain, the same duality: pointlike vs. diffuse, which we discovered in the spatial meaning of dendritic trees. It is important to keep both images in mind: (1) a sequence of spikes as a succession of individual events, each representing its own message well defined in time, and, (2) a sequence of spikes "read" by the receiver only in terms of the average frequency, calculated over long stretches of time.

References

4.1 Blinkov, S.M., Glezer, I.I.: The Human Brain in Figures and Tables. A quantitative handbook. New York: Plenum Press, Basic Books, Inc. Publ. 1968

4.2 Eccles, J.C.: The Physiology of Synapses. Berlin-Göttingen-Heidelberg-New York: Springer, 1964

4.3 Griesinger, W.: Die Pathologie und Therapie der psychischen Krankheiten. Stuttgart: Adolph Krabbe, 1861

4.4 Hodgkin, A.L.: The Conduction of the Nervous Impulse. Liverpool: Liverpool Univ. Press, 1964

4.5 Katz, B.: Nerve, Muscle and Synapse. New York-St. Louis-San Francisco: McGraw-Hill, 1966

4.6 Krafft-Ebing, R.V.: Lehrbuch der Psychiatrie. Stuttgart: Ferdinand Enke, 1897

4.7 Palay, S.L., Palade, G.E.: The fine structure of neurons. J. Biophys. Biochem. Cytol. *1*, 69–88 (1955)

5. How Accurately Are Brains Designed?*

It is surprising how little attention has been paid to the nervous system of arthropods and particularly to that of insects during the last decades which have otherwise produced such a copious neurological bibliography. These animals possess an extraordinarily complex and differentiated nervous system, and a fineness of structure that reaches the limits of the ultramicroscopic.   *Cajal and Sanchez [5.5]*

Most of the structure of a brain as we see it by macroscopic and microscopic observation is genetically determined. This conclusion may be reached simply from the observation that newborn, or even embryonic brains already have well-developed structures before the attached sense organs have ever received stimuli. No one seriously believes that we begin life as unstructured beings, as "tabulae rasae": clean slates on which only experience will leave marks. Yet, it is not to be doubted that some of the structure of the brain is formed during a learning phase, and probably embodies experience. There have been several claims in recent years of certain microscopic, and even macroscopic features of the brain developing in different ways under the influence of conditions imposed by the environment [5.8, 5.10]. On the whole, however, it is probably safe to say that memory traces have up to now escaped microscopic observation. What we see is inborn structure, or rather, if some of the histologic detail is due to learning, we do not know how to relate it to specific memory traces.

Defining the limits between inborn and acquired conditions of brain structure is not easy, especially since there is a third component that certainly also plays a part in the establishment of connections between neurons, namely, chance. This varies in importance according to one's philosophic outlook. The same people who, in order to simplify psychology, would like to see man and animals initially as clean slates, tend to reconcile the theoretical blankness with the undeniable existence of structure in newborn brains by considering these as products of chance.

---

* To Martin.

We can now approach the question of the role of randomness in brain anatomy by comparing the informational capacity of the genetic text (the upper limit of genetically dictated structure) with the amount of structure found in brain anatomy.

The amount of information passed on from parent to child through the germ cells can be computed if the length of the DNA thread is known. This is the giant molecule in which genetic information is contained as a chain of a large number of molecular subunits of four different sorts. Only the maximum amount of information that the germ cells can transfer, if the thread-like molecules were utilized to capacity, can be directly computed; not the information actually transferred, which is certainly considerably less. However that may be, the precision with which the structure of an organism is specified by the genes has its limits in the information capacity of the molecular thread. In humans the information capacity of the genetic material is said to be of the order of 10^{10} bits.

What information is contained there? Certainly all the detail that medical students learn in a thousand-page textbook of anatomy and in an equally long one of physiology. But this gets us hardly beyond the magnitude of 10^6 bits (not counting illustrations), from which we might draw the conclusion that our knowledge to date about the structure of the organism is quite poor. On the other hand, there is nothing in the textbook of anatomy about individual peculiarities, which also occupy some of the genetic information channel: the characteristic constitution of each individual's proteins, and the consequent variations of morphologic and other macroscopic characteristics of the individual, such as body build, color of the skin and hair, nose shape, possibly also individual variations of neural connections in the brain, etc.

If we ask how large a part of the genetic text is taken up by information about the structure of the nervous system, we may immediately be convinced that for a kilogram of brain more instructions are necessary than for the same amount of liver, or bone substance, skin, or muscle, because the brain has the least homogeneous structure. The liver, the lungs, muscles, skin, all organs in fact except the brain, have a periodic structure in which an elementary subunit, for example, a lobule of the liver, repeats itself almost identically. It is then enough for genetic inheritance that the structure of this elementary unit be specified along with the instruction to repeat it until a certain limit of size of the whole organ is reached. In anatomical textbooks, too, the chapter on the brain is much more voluminous than that on the liver, even if we have a rather thorough understanding of the structure of the liver down to the molecular level, while at present we can only give a very summary description of the feltwork of fibers in the brain. One has the impression that a well-developed neuroanatomy of the future will occupy at least as many pages as the entire anatomy of the rest of the body.

Besides these considerations, which are perhaps of interest to scientific publishers, the question arises as to whether the genetic text is at all sufficient to specify in detail the connections of the neurons in the brain. The answer to this question is certainly no, since the 10^{10} bits of the genetic code would be just sufficient to determine which of the 10^{10} neurons belong to the brain and which do not (a binary decision, a yes/no alternative per neuron) or which are to send an axon upward, which downward, but not sufficient to decide with which of the other neurons each neuron should make a synaptic connection.

We may draw two conclusions from this, both of which probably apply: (1) The pattern of the connections of neurons within the brain is only roughly determined by genetics, the details are the result of the individual's personal experience. Changes in the synaptic pattern, for example through a mechanism that creates stable connections between those neurons that are often active simultaneously or that disrupts the connections between those neurons that have no correlated activity, represent the most likely explanation for the phenomena called memory and learning. (2) The brain is also, like the liver or the skin, heavily redundant in its structure. Genetic information does not need to specify where each fiber should grow. Large fiber bundles that issue in an orderly array from a sense organ are distributed in the brain in an arrangement that mirrors the original array. For the establishment of such connections, an instruction is probably sufficient that proceeds much more summarily than if it directed each fiber to a particular address. The major part of a vertebrate brain, and also of an arthropod brain, has a cortex-like structure: a connecting scheme between input neurons in one level, and output neurons in another, is repeated almost identically over a wide surface. One can imagine that genetics contributes little more than the elementary coupling instruction in a narrow field — the rest is formed by repetition.

One thing, however, is certain. There are instances in which nerve tissue is constructed with absolute precision, in the sense that an exactly predictable connection is assigned to every single fiber. I know two examples of this in the visual system of the fly. The most impressive example is the projection of the retina onto the first visual ganglion, the lamina ganglionaris. The other example, within the same ganglion, is of special interest here since it provided the opportunity for observing pathology at the level of the connective scheme of individual fibers, i. e., an aberrant pattern of the weave in a few flies.

Projection of the Visual Field Onto the Lamina of the Fly[6]. The fly, like other insects, comes equipped with two large facet or compound eyes, which certainly play the main role in insect visual perception (Fig. 5.1). The term facet eye refers to the appearance of the surface, which is composed of a large number of "facets" — in the fly, about 3000 lenses on each side that project the optical input onto the same number of separate channels in which light is absorbed, transduced into chemical processes, and further into signals in a neural network. In contrast to the eyes of vertebrates, in which one single lens projects a picture onto a retina composed of a large number of light-sensitive elements (much like the situation in a photographic camera), the compound eye, to a first approximation, is an array of divergent tubes optically isolated from each other, each one seeing its own small part of the visual field. The advantage of this arrangement is that one can easily construct eyes that see all around, while the visual angle in the single-lens eye is necessarily reduced. The great disadvantage of the tubular eye (or facet eye) is its limited optical resolution, or to put it another way, its reduced light-gathering power. These two limitations are in fact related to each other. If we construct a compound eye by putting together a large number of very thin tubes, we obtain a good spatial discrimination of the visual field, but the single tube gets very

▶

FIGURE 5.1. Silver-stained section through part of the compound eye of the fly, from the surface to the first ganglion, the lamina ganglionaris (*lg*). The periodically repeating units of the compound eye are called ommatidia, the corresponding compartments or modules of the lamina are the neuroommatidia or "cartridges." The lenses of the cornea (*l*) together with the crystalline cones (*c*) form the dioptric apparatus of the eye. The focal plane of the system is at the level marked *f*, where the light-sensitive elements are arranged in the pattern of Figure 5.2. The photopigments are contained in the retinula cells between the levels f and b, the basal membrane. The 8 retinula cells of each ommatidium distribute their axons on several modules of the lamina (*a*) (cf. Figs. 5.3–5.6). The dark irregularly shaped structures that accompany the ommatidia between f and b are cells containing screening pigment. × 650

---

[6]   Braitenberg [5.2]; Horridge and Meinertzhagen [5.6]; Kirschfeld [5.7]; Vigier [5.11]

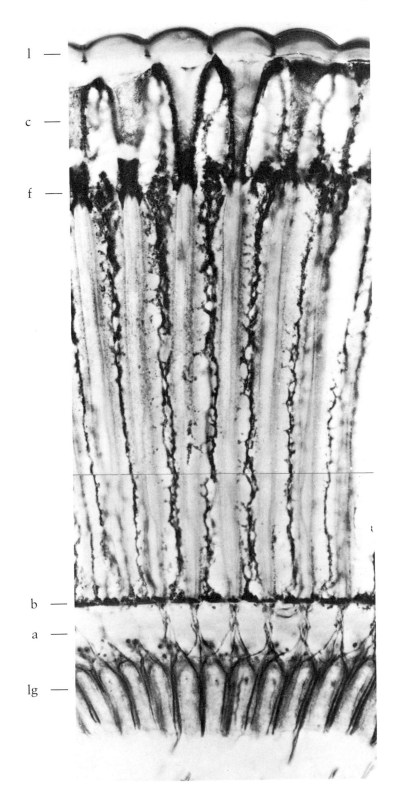

little light (technically speaking, "has a small aperture"). Contrarily, if the tubes are given a wide opening, then the fineness of the grain of the visual picture suffers. The fly eye with its 3000 facets (or ommatidia) on each side, is probably a good compromise between both demands. The sensitivity to light is surprisingly good; the resolution is, however, poor, since the angular separation between neighboring ommatidia is roughly 3°. Considering that the full moon measures about $1/2°$ in diameter, the fly sees the moon the way we see Mars with the naked eye: a minute dot in the sky, hopelessly beyond the optical resolution of our visual system.

Even more interesting is the discovery that behind each lens in the fly's eye there are not one, but seven light-sensitive elements, arranged in a regular though asymmetric array (Fig. 5.2). Was our notion of 6000 ommatidia as separate tubes, each one looking at only one spot in the sky, too hasty? Does the fly perhaps scan its surroundings with 6000×7 visual rays?

These questions can be answered by asking two further questions. The elements of the "retinula" (Fig. 5.2), as this arrangement of light detectors is called, only "see" separate regions of the visual field provided they are situated in or near the focal plane of the optical system. This seems to be the case, as we know from some experiments

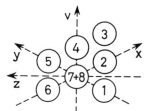

FIGURE 5.2. The retinula, i.e., the pattern of the seven light-sensitive elements in the focal plane of the ommatidium (f in Fig. 5.1). The pattern is that of the upper half of the right eye, seen from the outside. The arrow v points upward, z backward. x and y: the two oblique directions of the ommatidial array

►

FIGURE 5.3. Diagram illustrating the projection of the visual field onto the modules of the lamina ganglionaris (L) via the lenses (C) and the fibers of the retinula cells (R). Parallel rays are projected onto a set of 7 retinula cells (only 3 in the drawing) located in 7 different ommatidia, one in each ommatidium. The fibers of the corresponding retinula cells come together in one of the modules of the ganglion (black in the drawing)

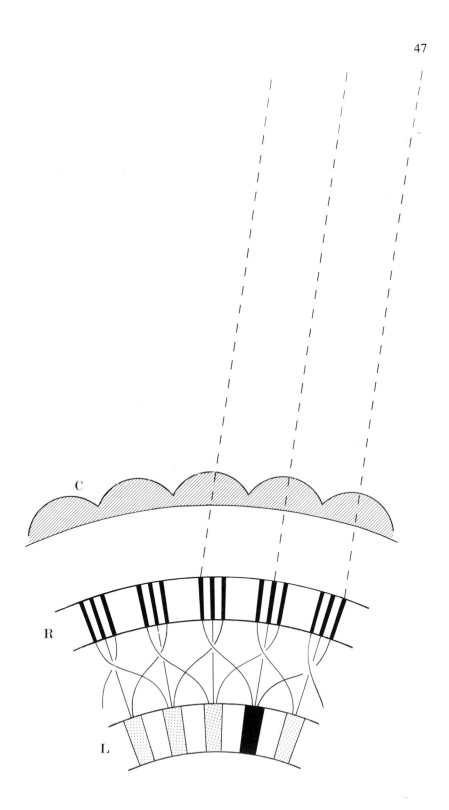

[5.1, 5.7] in which a flat cut shaved off from a fly's eye, including several ommatidia, was viewed through a microscope from within, i. e., in the same direction in which the fly looks through it. A distant, point-like light source makes individual elements of the retinula light up while the others remain in the dark. This proves the efficiency of the ommatidial lens as an imaging device: a section of the optical surroundings is actually broken down into single points by the seven elements of the retinula. The second question is, how large is the field of vision that belongs to a single retinula, and how do the seven visual rays of one retinula connect with the seven visual rays of each of the neighboring retinulas? The experimental answer is quite surprising [5.7]. It is derived partly from the foregoing experiment with the point-like light source and partly from the observation of the so-called pseudopupils. These are groups of facets of the fly's compound eye that, when illuminated from outside, appear darker, because they absorb more light than the other facets or, when illuminated from within, appear lighter than the others, because they convey light through the lenses of the eye directly into the lens of the microscope. Pseudopupils make it possible to identify those elements of the compound eye that look straight at the observer's eye. The answer is, the visual rays of a single ommatidium, corresponding to the seven elements of the retinula, are arranged exactly like the array of visual rays that we had initially supposed when we had attributed a single visual ray, a central ray to each ommatidium. The six peripheral visual rays (1–6 in Fig. 5.2) are each exactly parallel to the central visual ray of 6 other ommatidia, so that in all 7 visual rays of 7 different ommatidia look in the same direction: the central visual ray of one ommatidium, and one visual ray in each of 6 neighboring ommatidia. Because of the very small distance between neighboring ommatidia, the 7 parallel rays practically coincide. This means that at any given time 7 elements belonging to 7 different retinulas receive the same information from the environment.

This impressive result concerning the peripheral optics of the compound eye becomes interesting in connection with our neuroanatomical questions since it can be shown that the following proposition holds:

▶

FIGURE 5.4. Vertical section (parallel to the optical axis) through the fiber layer that connects the retina to the lamina of the fly. The bundles of retinula cell axons, which emerge at the base of each ommatidium (*arrows*) are twisted through 180° before they distribute their fibers onto different modules of the lamina. *R: retina; L:* lamina ganglionaris, *C:* "cartridges" of the lamina. Silver stain. × 1000

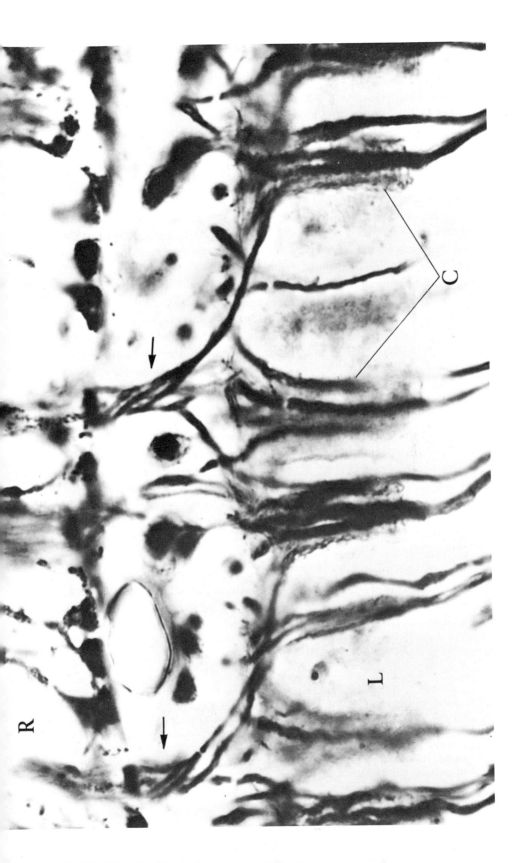

The 7 visual cells in 7 different ommatidia that see the same point of the visual field, send their fibers into one and the same compartment of the lamina ganglionaris [5.2].

All information from one of the 6000 points into which the visual field of the fly is subdivided, comes together in one little compartment of the ganglion. There are as many of these compartments as there are facets and ommatidia; in fact, they correspond one-to-one to the ommatidia of the eye and are therefore sometimes called neuro-ommatidia. The compound eye represents the optical environment on a screen of as many points as there are facets to the eye, just as the naive observation of the array of ommatidia had initially suggested.

To this, a few additional remarks: Every fiber stemming from an ommatidium must reach a point in the ganglion that deviates from the compartment directly below in the same direction and by as many units of the array as the corresponding visual ray deviates from the central visual ray of the ommatidium. This can easily be seen in Figure 5.3. Also, it is clear that the fiber bundle of each ommatidium has to be twisted around 180° to compensate the inversion of the image by the optical lens of the ommatidium. This means that the pattern formed by the neuro-ommatidia that are reached by the fibers of one ommatidium is the same as the pattern of the visual rays that issue forth from the ommatidium, if we think of them as projected on a plane. Consequently, it is also the same pattern as that of the elements in the retinula (Fig. 5.2), only inverted.

Figure 5.4 shows clearly the fulfillment of the first condition: that of the twist of the fiber bundle by 180°. The other condition, that of the repetition of the pattern of the retinula in the pattern of the distribution of the fibers onto the ganglion, seems at first glance not to be fulfilled. If we follow the fibers of one bundle on a flat section through this fiber layer (Fig. 5.5), we get the elongated distribution represented in Figure 5.6 a. This pattern becomes understandable only when the array of compartments of the lamina ganglionaris is stretched in a horizontal direction by a factor 3. Figure 5.6 a then goes over into Figure 5.6 b, which now exactly matches the pattern of the

▶

FIGURE 5.5. Tangential section through the fiber layer between the retina and the lamina of the fly. The section is perpendicular to that of Figure 14, at right angles to the axis of the optical system. However, because of the curvature of the eye, the angle between the section and the axis of the ommatidia is different in different regions of the micrograph. The striking regularity of this network is due to the repetition of the pattern illustrated in Figure 5.6. Silver stain. × 500

CHAMBLEE COLLEGE LIBRARY
LYONS, LUBBOCK, TEXAS

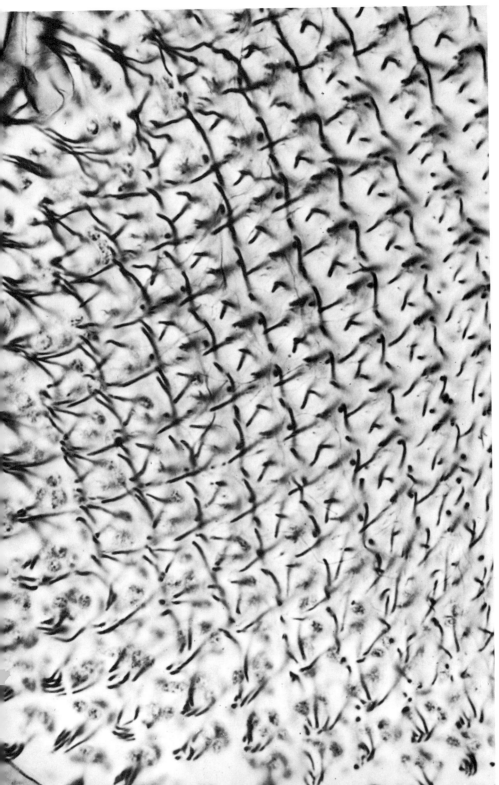

RIPON COLLEGE LIBRARY
RIPON, WISCONSIN 54971

retinula rotated 180°. Two things can be learned from this: first, the anatomical fact that the array of elements in the ganglia represents a metrically distorted projection of the visual field, because of the horizontal compression to ⅓ of the vertical dimension. (In fact, the ganglia are about 3 times as tall as they are wide, while the visual field of each eye measures 180° by 180°.) Second, we learn a trivial though surprising fact about the geometry of regular two-dimensional arrays. If one of the axes in a hexagonal array of dots is stretched to three times the original length, the array goes over into another, similar array with the same symmetry but with the distance between neighboring points enlarged by a factor of $\sqrt{3}$ and with the axes rotated 30°.

This interests us only marginally. Of central interest to us, however, is the precision with which the fiber distribution is accomplished (Fig. 5.5). Horridge and Meinertzhagen [5.6] went to the trouble to trace 650 single fibers on a series of sections on their path from the

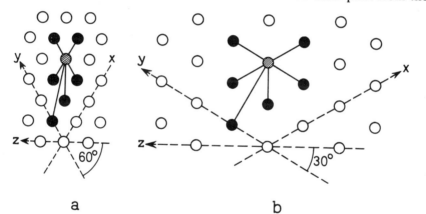

a   b

FIGURE 5.6. (a) Pattern of the distribution of the fibers from one ommatidium onto the modules of the lamina. (b) If the pattern is stretched threefold in the horizontal direction, it goes over into one that is identical with that of the retinula (Fig. 4.2), only rotated 180°. The geometric relation between a and b is consequence of the fact that the visual ganglia contain a foreshortened picture of the visual environment of the fly

FIGURE 5.7. Section through the lamina ganglionaris of the fly. The section is parallel to the axis of the ommatidia and so oriented that the structures shown lie on a vertical meridian of the fly's head. At the lower margin of the ganglion one can see fibers *(arrows)* that connect neighboring modules ("cartridges"). Compare Figure 5.8. *L:* lamina ganglionaris; *a:* fibers between the retina and the lamina; *b:* fibers between the lamina and the medulla. Silver stain. × 1200

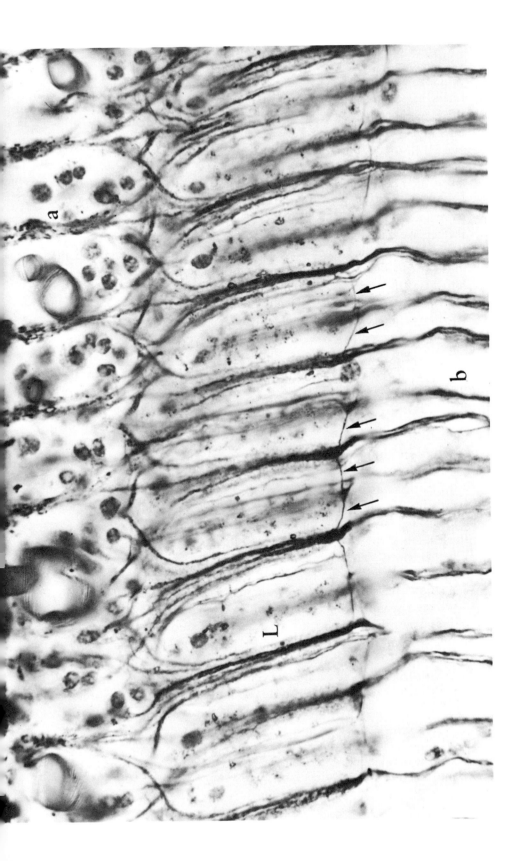

retina to the lamina ganglionaris. They confirmed that none of the
fibers missed the address appointed them by the rule given above.
What mechanisms guide the growth of the fibers is a question that we
intentionally do not want to discuss here. If one looks at Figure 5.5, it
will be clear that the idea which was occasionally put forth, that gradients of concentration of certain substances in different directions
lead each fiber to a particular point in the tissue, will be of little serv-
ice to us. The system of concentration gradients would have to be so
complicated that its effectiveness as an explanation would be lost.
Rather, we gain the impression that the bundles growing out of the
ommatidia contain in themselves the key to the distribution of fibers
in the net and do not have to wait for instructions from the structures
into which they grow. This is particularly clear in the middle section of
the fly's eye where, at the so-called equator, the fibers of the retinulas, mirror images of each other in the upper and lower half of the
eye, come together. Here each bundle behaves exactly as predicted by
our rule (the convergence of signals from one point of the visual field
onto one compartment of the ganglion) even in the region where the
fibers from the northern and from the southern retinulas, mirror symmetric to each other, overlap.

In any case, this example shows that in certain places, at least in
the nervous system of insects, there exists a wiring that is so precise
that there is no room for chance.

The *second example* [5.3, 5.4, 5.9] refers to the network
represented in Figures 5.7, 5.8 and 5.9, Figures 5.7 and 5.8 show the
normal anatomy. At the lower edge of the lamina ganglionaris two
small fibers come out of each of the bundles that correspond to the
"compartments" already mentioned (Fig. 5.7). The fibers reach two
neighboring bundles, one above and to the rear, and the other below
and to the rear in the array of compartments (Fig. 5.8) and there
make their synaptic connections. The electron microscope shows that
these fibers probably mediate reciprocal interactions between neighboring compartments, since the connections are made by pairs of synapses in opposite directions. In the normal fly this net has a regular
weave. In one series of flies, however, white-eyed mutants, which ap-
peared in the breed of our institute, we found, to our surprise, a net-

▶

FIGURE 5.8. Flat cut through the network formed by the fibers marked
with arrows on Figure 5.7. The fibers run from each module of the ganglion to two neighboring modules in the two oblique directions of the
array. The arrow z points backward. Silver stain. × 1200

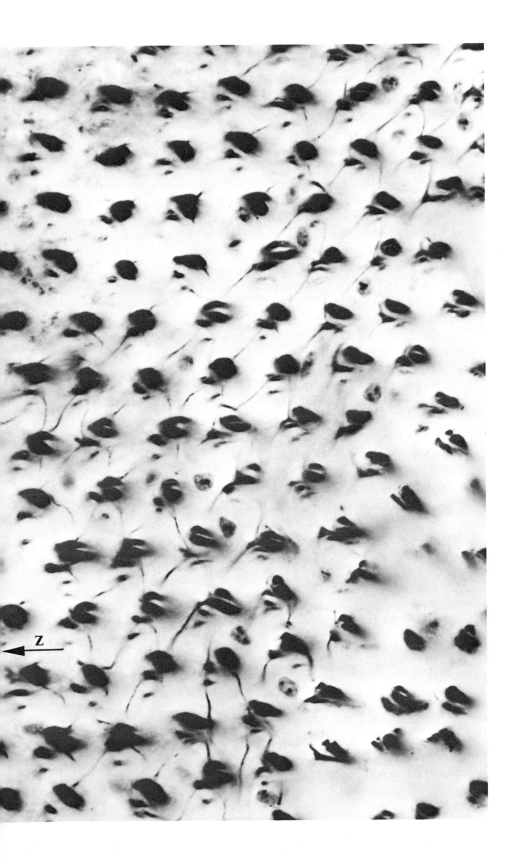

work that deviates from that of the normal fly (Fig. 5.9). In addition to the two fibers leading above and to the rear there was an additional small fiber in many meshes that led directly to the neighboring bundle at the rear. We have not yet been able to discover the conditions under which this variation of the wiring appears. It does not seem to be connected merely with the genetic mutation manifested in the pigmentless eyes, since in many other white-eyed flies that were later examined, we could not find the aberrant wiring. The group of white-eyed flies that had the extra fiber could perhaps have been subjected to abnormal conditions during their development (involving temperature, humidity, light, food, etc.); the abnormal anatomy could have been determined, at least in part, by these external influences. However this may be, the case is interesting as an example of brain pathology at the level of the detailed wiring of neurons. In man, missing fiber bundles, poor subdivision of the cerebral gray matter, or similar gross defects have been observed in cases of mental debility and other psychic disorders, but until now nothing as fine as a change in the wiring scheme of single meshes in a neural network has been shown. The minute variations in the wiring in our white-eyed flies are as little apparent in the gross anatomical picture of the fly brain as the weaving mistakes perhaps existing in the brains of humans with inherited psychoses, for which an anatomical basis has yet to be found. Up to now, human brain pathology has been oriented mainly toward the changes apparent in the cell body. The study of fiber connections has been neglected by pathologists, perhaps due to the considerable technical problems involved.

References

5.1   Autrum, H. J., Wiedemann, I.: Versuche über den Strahlengang im Insektenauge (Appositionsauge). Z. Naturforsch. *17b*, 480–482 (1962)
5.2   Braitenberg, V.: Patterns of projection in the visual system of the fly. I. Retina-lamina projections. Exptl. Brain Res. *3*, 271–298 (1967)
5.3   Braitenberg, V.: The anatomical substratum of visual perception in flies. A sketch of the visual ganglia. Rendiconti S. I. F. XLIII, Reichardt, W. (ed.) London-New York: Academic Press, 1969, pp. 328–340

▶

FIGURE 5.9. The same fibers as in Figure 5.8, but with a pathologic variation. Besides the two fibers running from each module to the two neighbors behind and above and behind and below, in some instances (*arrows*) *there is a third branch running toward the module directly behind. z:* arrow pointing backward. × 1000

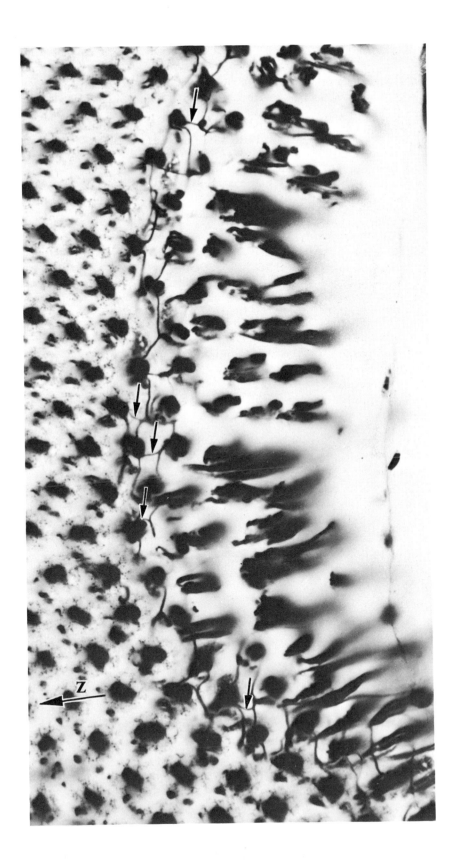

5.4   Braitenberg, V., Debbage, P.: A regular net of reciprocal synapses in the visual system of the fly, *Musca domestica*. J. Comp. Physiol. *90*, 25–31 (1974)

5.5   Cajal, S. R., Sanchez, D.: Contribucion al conocimiento de los centros nerviosos de los insectos. Parte 1. Retina y centros opticos. Trab. Lab. Invest. Biol. Univ. Madr. *13*, 1–168 (1915)

5.6   Horridge, G. A., Meinertzhagen, I. A.: The accuracy of the pattern of connexions of the first- and second-order neurons of the visual system of *Calliphora*. Proc. Roy. Soc. Lond. Ser. B *175*, 69–82 (1970)

5.7   Kirschfeld, K.: Die Projektion der optischen Umwelt auf das Raster der Rhabdomere im Komplexauge von Musca. Exptl. Brain Res. *3*, 248–270 (1967)

5.8   Rosenzweig, M. R., Bennett, E. L., Diamond, M. C.: Brain changes in response to experience. Sci. Amer. *226/2*, 22 (1972)

5.9   Strausfeld, N. J., Braitenberg, V.: The compound eye of the fly (*Musca domestica*): connections between the cartridges of the lamina ganglionaris. Z. vergl. Physiol. *70*, 95–104 (1970)

5.10 Valverde, F.: Apical dendritic spines of the visual cortex and light deprivation in the mouse. Exptl. Brain Res. *3*, 337–352 (1967)

5.11 Vigier, P.: Mécanisme de la synthèse des impressions lumineuses recueillies par les yeux composés des Diptères. C. R. Acad. Sci. Paris 122–124 (1907)

6. Neuroanatomical Invariants: Analysis of the Cerebellar Cortex*

> *Symmetry, as wide or as narrow as you may define its meaning, is one idea by which man through the ages has tried to comprehend and create order, beauty, and perfection.* Hermann Weyl [6.12]

Transformation and Invariance

In the previous chapter we tried to answer the question concerning the level of precision at which the wiring of nerve nets is defined by considering two special cases. The question of constancy has a more general aspect. I will first introduce it in a philosophical way, borrowing some concepts from geometry, which will then guide us in an approach to that most spectacular structure of the vertebrate brain, the cerebellar cortex.

When we talk about a certain structure, we must first be able to recognize what we have in mind irrespective of all the variations of its appearance. This is a familiar situation when we think of the accidental, random variations (the so-called noise) that affect every repetition of a constant blueprint: we can never draw exactly the same triangle twice on the blackboard, yet we still keep talking about "the triangle," just as my friend is never exactly the same from one day to the next and is still constantly my friend. It is less trivial and more interesting to consider systematic variations. Thus I may decide that "a family resemblance" is the face I have in mind after I have systematically observed all the faces of the members of that clan. The discovery of constant features in systematic variations is a fundamental, powerful procedure: it is the first step in the definition of "things" that safeguards us from wasting our time in considerations of accidental, nonessential aspects. This idea becomes more precise in geometry. Different kinds of properties of geometric objects can be defined by indicating the transformations of the space in which the objects are embedded, which leave these properties unchanged ("invariant"). If we imagine a plane as a rubber membrane that we can stretch in any way, the so-called topologic properties of shapes drawn on the plane

---

* Dedicated to Nello.

will be preserved while other properties, which we call metric, will not be preserved. An 8 drawn on a rubber membrane will keep its form no matter how it is distorted, if by its form we mean: a shape with two holes. The two holes belong to the topologic characteristics of the image of the number 8. The peculiarity that the upper loop of the 8 is smaller than the lower can be easily changed by a distortion of the substrate and does not belong to the topologic description. In this sense a particular geometry is determined by the set of operations that can be carried out on a class of figures without changing the relevant properties. In one kind of geometry the properties of figures are not changed, regardless of the extent to which they are enlarged, rotated, or shifted; in another kind, the relevant properties are not changed even if one looks at their silhouettes projected on a plane by a point-like light source, etc.

Of what use is this in brain anatomy? One can hope by this means to escape the uncertainty that strikes us at the very beginning when we try to understand the meaning of a complex structure of nerve fibers: we do not know which geometric characteristics of the structure are worth pointing out, which are due to chance, and which are irrelevant because they are too general. If there is the possibility of following the same structure through some natural variation, one can consider those aspects of the structure that remain invariant throughout all transformations as being the essentially relevant ones. In analogy to geometry, we will obtain the structural plan at different levels of abstraction depending on the set of transformations considered.

What kinds of transformation are at our disposal if we are looking for the invariants in the structure of a central nervous organ?

First, the variation of a piece of nerve tissue from individual to individual of the same species. Comparison is always possible if we can recognize a certain organ of the brain in different individuals of the same species by virtue of its position relative to other parts of the brain, or by virtue of particular fiber bundles with which it is connected. Individual differences in the number, size, or arrangement of nerve elements can always be found by exact quantitative, microscopic analysis. Even in the unusually regular nerve nets of the visual system of the fly, interindividual variations in the number of meshes, thickness of fibers, and relative position of fibers at the crossing points can easily be found. What, in both cases, (normally) remains constant is the connecting scheme given in Figures 5.6 and 5.8, respectively. It is obtained as the invariant pattern on the background of individual variation, whatever the cause of the variation. We may suppose that those structural properties of a piece of nerve tissue that are interindividually constant correspond to the genetically determined information.

This assertion calls for two comments. By this method, we cannot ascertain the total genetic information pertaining to a certain nerve structure, but only the part that is common to the whole species. From genetics and evolution theory we know that part of the genetic blueprint is individually variable and is certainly co-responsible for the observed anatomical variety. The other difficulty in trying to infer genetic information from anatomy is the following. As long as we do not have better knowledge of the growth mechanisms of nerve tissue, it is difficult to estimate whether what we observe in the microscope is genetically determined to the last detail, or is rather the general consequence of a developmental process. Because of the specificity of some neuronal connections, we might be tempted to suppose that there is more genetic information than really necessary if some kind of constructional rule is responsible for a part of the regularity of the nerve net (the tendency of cells to distribute themselves evenly in the available space, to produce cell processes with radial symmetry, perhaps a certain temporal sequence in the outgrowths of different cell processes, etc.).

Second, we can often observe local structural variations within a piece of nerve tissue that seems at first glance to have a uniform structure. These variations can be understood as modifications of a basic plan. The basic plan can be recognized as the description that remains invariant, irrespective of local variation.

The most impressive example of a structural scheme realized in an unbelievably large number of variations is the cerebral cortex of man. The net is woven out of a small number of neuronal types. The size of the neurons, the length and thickness of their extensions, and the thickness of the layers of the cortex in which their cell bodies are situated are, however, very different from area to area. Apparently, the fundamental operation for which the cerebral cortex is responsible, occurs in different ways when it is applied to the visual, acoustic, or tactile input or when it is carried out in the region where the motor output arises, or at the place whose destruction results in incapacity of speech. If we wanted to know the nature of the computation carried out in the cortex, a problem to which we shall return in the last chapter, we would have to refer to the invariant, basic pattern underlying the local "areal" variation. We should not, however, in an attempt to define the basic structure of the cerebral cortex miss the opportunity provided by a further variation that is available for the discovery of invariants, namely:

Third: the variations of a neurologic mechanism in different kinds of animals. Sometimes we can easily recognize homologous parts of the brain in very different, only distantly related animal species such as frog and man. In many cases the homology is perfectly clear even though it may not always be easy to define the criteria used in the identification. In the olfactory bulb, a structure common to all vertebrates, the so-called olfactory glomeruli, characteristic little spherical knots in which the primary fibers of the sense of smell connect with second order neurons, are a constant fixture. They are a good reason for the assumption that in fish, batrachians, reptiles, birds, and mammals the olfactory bulb is merely a modification of a well-established, primal olfactory apparatus. The first, second, and third visual ganglia can be identified without difficulty in all species of insects; even in other arthropods, such as isopods and crabs, the similarity to insects in the arrangement and in the structure of these ganglia is such that the various levels of the visual system of all arthropods can be well compared. That these structures have much in common even in animals that have very different ways of living (flying, swimming, crawling, living in light or shadow, aggressive or shy) indicates that there must be a common function that has been adapted to the requirements of the different species.

Fourth, particularly in the so-called cortices consisting of nervous tissue that is spread out in large plates, one can observe folds, distortions, and bulges that are related to the necessity of fitting a large surface into a relatively small skull. The human cortex consists, for example, of two pieces, each the size of a handkerchief. The cerebellum in man has the shape and size of a long, tattered scarf about 17 cm wide and 1.20 m long. The folding of these structures distorts some measurements and leaves others invariant. The example of the cerebellar cortex, in comparison to the cerebral cortex, will show how the structural invariants connected with the folding can be interpreted as a consequence of a special functional principle that distinguishes the cerebellum from other parts of the nervous system.

Fifth, a series of concepts such as mirror-reflection, translation, rotation can be borrowed from geometry: operations that define different types of symmetry of the figures to which they are applied, depending on whether or not they lead to a result that is identical to the original figures. Mirror symmetry, translational symmetry, radial symmetry, and other types can be thus defined and applied to various kinds of neural tissues.

Geometricians should not be disturbed by the fact that the structures in the brains are neither ideal geometric structures, nor quasi-geometric ones like crystals. When we talk about symmetry as the group of transformations that leave figures unchanged, when we say, for example, that a mirror in the median plane of the body makes the right hemisphere of the brain identical to the left, then we merely mean that a brain anatomist employing his usual methods cannot tell from a photograph whether it represents the right or the left half of a histologic preparation of the brain. In neuroanatomy, "that-which-a-brain-anatomist-cannot-distinguish" takes the place of "identical" in the geometric definition. The language of geometry is convenient and fruitful in this pragmatic application.

Analysis of the Cerebellum[7]

> The cerebellum seems to have very little to do with higher psychic activity.
>> Griesinger, 1861 [6.7], not contradicted since

> We must concede that we know practically nothing about the events that take place between the arrival of the afferent signals and the response of the Purkinje neurons or the modulation of their discharge.
>> Dow and Moruzzi, 1958 [6.4]

> It is generally believed that in some way the cerebellum functions as a type of computer.
>> Eccles, Ito and Szentágothai, 1967 [6.5]

In different animal species, the cerebellum varies a great deal in size both absolutely and relative to the rest of the brain. It is constant, however, in its position in relation to other parts of the brain, even though it appears now as a modest plate wedged between midbrain and rhombencephalon, as in the frog, now as an imposing growth rooted in the same place, as in humans, and particularly impressive in the electric fish, *Gnathonemus*. A section through the cerebellum shows in every case a continuous, sometimes richly folded plate of uniform structure covering the surface of the organ, the so-called cerebellar cortex, to which a large bundle of fibers is attached which connects it in its entire width in both directions with other parts of the brain.

We will now try to collect some propositions that are valid for the cerebella of all vertebrates in so far as their histology is known. In formulating such a set of invariants of cerebellar structure, certain aspects will fall by the wayside. For example, cell types that are present in the cerebellum of some species of animals, but not in all, evidently are not part of the structure, and therefore, not part of the function of the cerebellum in its most general formulation. The general plan of the connections within the cerebellar cortex that remains constant in a review of all animal species shall serve as basis for our thoughts on the function of this piece of nerve tissue (Fig. 6.1).

1. As in the other pieces of gray substance spread out in sheets,

---

[7] Braitenberg [6.1], Braitenberg and Atwood [6.2]; Braitenberg and Onesto [6.3], Eccles et al. [6.5]; Llinas (ed.) [6.8]

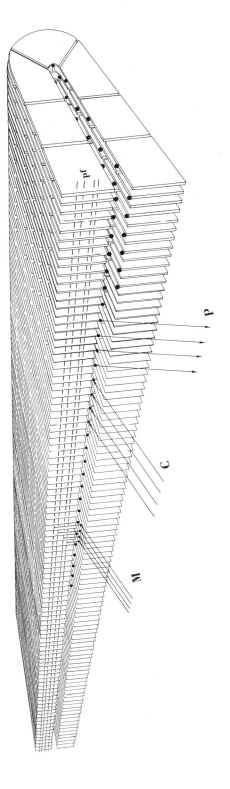

FIGURE 6.1. Diagrammatic view of a piece of the cerebellar cortex, folded in the shape of the typical cerebellar convolution, the so-called folium. The dendritic trees of the Purkinje cells are represented as flat square boxes. The regularity of their arrangement, but not the rigor of their parallel orientation, is exaggerated in the drawing. The cell bodies of the Purkinje cells are represented as large black dots, those of some granular cells as small dots. The arrows P represent the axons of some Purkinje cells, the arrows C are the climbing fibers belonging to some other Purkinje cells and the arrows M are the mossy fibers contacting some granular cells. The axons of the granular cells divide to form the parallel fibers, pf, which travel through a large number of Purkinje-cell dendritic trees. Other neuronal elements of the cerebellar cortex that may not belong to the standard equipment of the cerebellum of all vertebrate species, are not included in the drawing

the so-called cortices, the plan of the arrangement of different neuronal types in different layers and the pattern of their connections are repeated with great constancy over the whole surface.

At variance with the situation in the cerebral cortex, however, where the connections are arranged in all directions of the cortical plane, the fibers in the cerebellar cortex run almost exclusively in two perpendicular directions, longitudinally and transversely. The two sets of fibers are also very different in type. Very different histologic pictures are obtained by sectioning the cerebellar cortex in planes parallel or perpendicular to the long axis of the animal (in both cases perpendicular to the cortical plane: so-called vertical sections. Note that we have to disregard the folding, imagining the cerebellar cortex as if ironed out into a plane in order to apply this terminology). Very different fiber populations are responsible for the functional interactions of the neurons in the two directions of the cortical sheet.

In contrast to the cerebellar cortex, if we were to show a histologic preparation of the cerebral cortex to a fellow neuroanatomist he would not be able to tell in which direction the section was oriented. He could of course determine the angle between the plane of the section and the plane of the cortex, but not the orientation in the cortical plane (Fig. 6.2). As far as the function of the cerebral cortex is concerned, from the homogeneity of the network in all directions of the plane, one could conclude that the functional interactions are also the same in all directions and that the effect of one neuron upon another depends only on the distance and not on their relative positions. If one likes geometry, one can express the structural types of both cortices, the cerebral and the cerebellar cortex, more abstractly by indicating the geometric operations that transform the structure into an indistinguishable one. In the case of the cerebral cortex it is any shift in any direction (I cannot tell from which place in the cerebral cortex a particular preparation has been taken), and, in addition, the rotation around the vertical axis (I cannot determine in which direction the

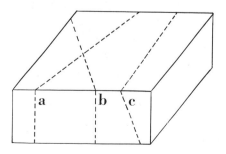

FIGURE 6.2. Various cuts through a cortex. *a* and *b*, vertical cuts. They would be indistinguishable in the cerebral cortex, but might yield entirely different histologic pictures in the cerebellar cortex. *c*, oblique cut, always distinguishable from a or b

section was made.) In the case of the cerebellar cortex it is the shift of a certain length (and its multiples) in one direction, and of a different length (and its multiples) in the direction perpendicular to it (this is somewhat idealized since the cerebellar cortex is not strictly periodic). Rotation around a vertical axis does not belong to the operations that lead to an identical structure in the case of the cerebellum. Only a special kind of rotation, that of 180°, transforms the structure of the cerebellar cortex into itself: there are planes of mirror symmetry, both longitudinal as well as transverse ones.

2. The fibers that carry the output from the cerebellar cortex, the only ones that relay signals from the cerebellum to other parts of the nervous system, originate in a particular kind of neuron, the so-called Purkinje cells. These are distinguished by a richly branching dendritic tree, whose branches do not grow out in all directions as in an oak tree, but mainly in a plane perpendicular to the transverse direction in a manner reminiscent of fruit trees trained to grow up against the walls of houses. If one cuts the cerebellar cortex longitudinally, in so-called sagittal sections, the Purkinje-cell dendritic trees (in man) appear about 10 times as wide as when one looks at them in transversely cut preparations, in so-called frontal sections. There are about 15 million Purkinje cells in man.

3. The Purkinje cells are embedded in a thick felt of fibers that covers the whole cerebellar cortex forming the so-called molecular layer. (The name recalls in a touching fashion an age when one assumed that many pieces of gray matter were homogeneous down to the molecular level, because fine nerve fibers could not yet be histologically demonstrated and few cell nuclei could be seen there.) The major portion of this felt consists of very thin fibers a few millimeters long, all running in the same direction, perpendicular to the long axis of the animal, and perpendicular to the plane of the flat dendritic trees of the Purkinje cells. In smaller cerebella, for example in the frog, each one of these so-called parallel fibers reaches from the right to the left edge of the cerebellar cortex. In the more highly developed cerebella, for example in man, they are shorter than the width of the cerebellum and are staggered in all possible relative positions in the fiber felt. On closer inspection each parallel fiber reveals itself as the cross bar of the T-shaped branching of one of the fibers rising up from below the molecular layer. These originate in small neurons called granular cells of which there are a great number, in man between 10^{10} and 10^{11} in the whole cerebellum. This order of magnitude is often taken as the number of all neurons in man and is used in estimating

the lattice formed by the different neuronal populations of the molecular layer, in the transverse direction, the direction of the parallel fibers. Folds perpendicular to this, parallel to the longitudinal axis of the animal, are apparently avoided in the construction of the cerebellum, as if it were important to keep parallel fibers unbent and to keep the planes of the dentric trees of neighboring Purkinje cells always as parallel as possible to each other.

In contrast to other folded planar brain structures, which look like the surface of a walnut, or like a carelessly wrinkled cloth (for example, the cerebral cortex of larger mammals, the olivary nucleus of primates, the dentate nucleus), this parallel folding is a particularly striking characteristic of the cerebellar cortex. How may we interpret the folding of cortex-like structures, and how can we explain that in closely related species the same organ makes its appearance now as a smooth plate, and now as a folded structure? When there is such a difference, it is striking that the folding makes its appearance in the larger of two related species. If one had to design an enlarged version of a small monkey, one evidently could not simply copy the whole organism on a larger scale, just as an ocean liner cannot be just a larger edition of a fisherman's skiff. One of the reasons for this is that oars cannot be enlarged proportionally, since their size must maintain a certain relation to particles of constant size, namely to the people by whom they will be handled.

It seems that the thickness of cortices of animals of different sizes remains fairly constant: evidently the thickness is connected with the fundamental operation that takes place there. The increase in size of the cortex of larger animals is achieved mainly through an increase of the surface extension. If one assumes that the number of problems for which the cortex is responsible increases with the volume of the animal, or with the third power of the linear dimensions, a true-to-scale enlargement of the surface of the cortex, which goes with the second power of the linear dimensions, would not be enough. In large animals the cortex has to be folded.

I will now try to derive a few propositions about the function of the cerebellum from the foregoing collection of anatomical facts.

The same fundamental operation is carried out at all points of the cerebellar cortex. This follows simply from the continuous and uniform structure of the neuronal network. The uniformity of the cerebellar operation is astonishing, since certain areas of the cerebellum in mammals have something to do with the maintainance of equilibrium in standing upright or walking, and other areas more with the control of delicate movements in the extremities. This can be concluded from the different consequences of lesions to the various parts of the cerebellum. Also, the projections from different regions of the brain and spinal cord onto the cerebellum through climbing fibers and mossy fibers reveal complicated situations that are not easily interpreted. Different parts of the cerebellum receive their fibers from different regions of the nervous system, with partial overlap of the projection areas. The entirely different kinds of information that are assembled there, and the different scopes that the elaboration of the information in the cerebellar network serves (in one case the control of rapid voluntary movements, in another, the distribution of muscular tensions necessary for a stable upright posture, etc.) notwithstanding, the same trick of computation is apparently employed.

Certainly of importance in this connection is the fact that the cerebellar structure is not interrupted in the midline. The fiber felt of the parallel fibers and the rows of Purkinje cells continue across the midline without showing any singularity there. One cannot tell from a histologic section through the cerebellar cortex whether it includes parts of the right and left halves of the cerebellum, or whether it is just from one side. Where the cerebellum does show fissures that divide it (not completely) into one central and two lateral strips, a situation found in the posterior section of the cerebellum of all mammals, the fissures never lie on the midline, but always laterally to it. In the middle there is always a long uninterrupted ribbon of the cerebellar cortex reaching from the anterior to the posterior end of the cerebellum, the so-called cerebellar vermis.

This continuity over the midline distinguishes the cerebellum from the other parts of the brain, which almost without exception come in symmetric pairs, one right and one left. (Another exception is the small interpeduncular nucleus in the brainstem of many vertebrates whose structure is reminiscent of the cerebellum in other respects as well.) While evidently in many other functional contexts the brain steers the behavior, as it were, with two symmetric reins (think of an animal following a path, turning toward or away from an object, etc.), the cerebellum functions in a fashion in which the boundary between right and left is blurred. In the cerebellar cortex, whose right and left halves correspond to the right and left halves of the body, and therefore also to the right and left halves of the environment, two signals that stem from different places in one half of the body interact with each other in the same way as two signals from the two sides of the body that reach the cerebellum on either side of the midline, provided that they have the same relative position in the cerebellar cortex.

It is tempting to relate this structural continuity to the role the cerebellum plays in preserving equilibrium. If our body is in an erect position, we prevent ourselves from falling to the left or right by pitting the weights of both halves of the body against each other. This is done by changing the leverage upon which the various masses act, e. g., by changing the position of the arms. We do the same when the body is in a slanting position, for example, when we stand on one leg with the other off the ground. Again, balance is preserved by playing parts of the body masses against each other, but this time, not the left half against the right half, but a different distribution, depending upon the position. An organ that is to do this must be able to perform the same operations between right and left as within each half. If both sides of the body were attached to both halves of such an organ, fiber connections between right and left would not be expected to be different from those within each side, which is the case in the cerebellum. For the present, this thought cannot be developed beyond the identification of the same type of symmetry in a postulated function and in the observed structure of a nerve net. Thus far we have only a vague idea of the processes that are at the basis of the astonishing performances of equilibrium in animals while standing, running, swimming, and flying.

A second, general, and somewhat vague reflection on symmetry concerns the totally different fiber connections in the two directions of the cerebellar cortex (anteroposterior and transverse). Evidently, the cerebellar cortex cannot be considered as a two-dimensional continuum upon which two-dimensional sensory fields are homogeneously represented, as in the cerebral cortex, the retina, or the tectum of lower vertebrates: the visual field on the retina, the two-dimensional continuum of directions of motion on the motor cortex, etc. In the plane of the cerebellar cortex, the direction of the parallel fibers and the direction of the fibers perpendicular to these evidently correspond to entirely different variables in the space in which the cerebellar functions take place. It is probably misleading to draw little men (homunculi) on the map of the cerebellar cortex (as on the map of the cerebral cortex, where it is justified) in order to show to which parts of the body the corresponding regions of the cerebellar cortex are connected. At least the little men in the cerebellar map ought to be striped to remind us that the computation that occurs in the direction of the stripes is certainly entirely different from the one in the perpendicular direction. The projection of the environment (and the projection of other parts of the brain and body) on the cerebellar cortex, is certainly not to be understood as a homogeneous two-dimensional representation, but rather as the projection of different magnitudes on two one-dimensional systems that are arranged perpendicular to each other. We must try to guess what magnitudes are involved here.

We will turn our attention now to the peculiar behavior of the cerebellar cortex in regard to folding. Here two facts are particularly striking in comparison to the cerebral cortex: (1) the lack of folds in the longitudinal direction; (2) the constant thickness of the molecular layer: the bulging and stretching that accompanies the folding is all at the expense of the granular layer and leaves the molecular layer invariant.

It appears from this that in the molecular layer the folding not only respects the neighborhood relationships of the elements, but also keeps certain distances constant. This is quite different in the cerebral cortex. None of the layers there has a similar exceptional position. In the depth of the furrows, the deep layers are stretched and are correspondingly thinner, while the upper layers are bulging and thicker. The situation is reversed on the crest of the convolutions, where the surface of the cortex is convex. In the cerebral cortex what matters seems to be only the scheme of the connections of the elements, not the distance between them: the distortions that arise because of folding evidently have no bearing on the function, unless we want to ascribe to the cerebral cortex entirely different functions depending on whether it lies on the crest of a convolution or in the depth of a furrow. Something similar can certainly be said of the granular layer of the cerebellar cortex, which is much thicker below the convex folds of the cerebellar cortex than in the valleys of the convolutions. It seems as if this layer had only to preserve a certain volumetric relation to the corresponding sections of the molecular layer, while it does not seem to matter in what relative positions the granules are to each other. The molecular layer is entirely different: from its constant thickness, we may conclude that the distances between its elements play an essential part included in the computation for which it is responsible.

This thought becomes more precise when we think of the lack of folds in the longitudinal direction that is so striking in the cerebellum. Such folds would cause the planes of the flat ramifications of the Purkinje cell-dendrites to lean against each other, and the length of the parallel fiber pathways between one Purkinje cell and the next would depend on the height in the molecular layer. It seems, then, that in the cerebellar cortex it is important to preserve the distances mainly in one of the two main directions, in the transverse direction in which the parallel fibers run.

Now that our suspicion has fallen upon the transverse direction of the cerebellar cortex, upon the direction of the parallel fibers, we must ask ourselves what reason might there be for each signal in the parallel fiber system to be smeared over long distances, each parallel fiber transmitting the message to hundreds of Purkinje cells one after the other? Why the divergent transmission from each fiber to so many channels? If one were interested in multiplying signals, could that not be done more easily by ramification of the fibers, as occurs in many other parts of the brain?

The answer that comes to mind is this: although it is the same signal that arrives to a long row of Purkinje cells along a parallel fiber, it does not arrive at the same time at the different Purkinje cells. The running time of the impulses in the parallel fibers is certainly longer, the more distant the dendritic tree that receives them is situated from the branching point of the parallel fibers. A rapid calculation shows that, with a speed of conduction of a few decimeters per second, a maximal delay of a few milliseconds can be generated by each parallel fiber. The difference in the time of arrival of signals between neighboring Purkinje cell trees turns out to be about a tenth of a millisecond. Before we ask ourselves what significance these small time intervals might have in the information processing of the brain, we would like to try to illuminate the structural characteristics of the cerebellum, which we have previously assembled, with the newly won concept of the cerebellar cortex as a timing organ.

I maintain that with this thought of the cerebellar cortex as a clock in the millisecond range, all essential peculiarities of the cerebellar structure can be explained. We suddenly understand why the dendritic trees of the Purkinje cells are so flat: if the transverse direction in the molecular layer represents time, then a flat dendritic tree set perpendicular to it means a well-defined point in time. A synchronized wave of excitation in the molecular level, perhaps generated by signals in a group of closely neighboring granular cells, would arrive at a later point in time synchronously at a particular Purkinje cell. We understand also why the planes of these flat dendritic trees are held so strictly parallel to each other, a fact that we learned from the absence of folding in the longitudinal direction. This is to guarantee that a front of excitation is not dispersed on its way as it travels from one Purkinje cell to the next in a row. We can also find an argument for the multitude of parallel fibers based on their thinness. This is necessary in order to generate the desired delays without having to use overly long fibers: the speed of conduction is approximately proportionate to the cross section of the fibers. It could be, however, that such thin fibers generate only a very minor quantity of excitation, too little, perhaps, to activate a Purkinje cell. The multitude of parallel fibers that are all approximately in the same position of the cerebellar cortex, and therefore receive approximately the same mossy fiber input and connect with the same Purkinje cells, could be an answer to this problem. One can now assign a function also to the climbing fibers that were at first a riddle because of their one-to-one connection with the Purkinje cells. What is gained by switching from one system of several million fibers to another one with as many neurons, when each fiber in the new system at best can transfer the information that corresponds to a fiber in the old system? According to our concept, the climbing fibers are assigned the role of "setting" single Purkinje cells of the cerebellar clock. We may imagine different uses of such an arrangement in the following contexts:

1. A clock can serve as an alarm clock if one sets it to a future time at which one would like to receive a signal. This is done by marking a place on the clock, which, when reached by the hand, emits a signal. The marking of a place in the cerebellar cortex can be imagined as follows: the climbing fibers, in a restricted region of the molecular layer, activate several Purkinje cells so that a signal arriving through the parallel fibers meets with changed conditions at that place. What kind of interaction takes place between the signals in the mossy fiber parallel system on the one hand, and the climbing fiber system on the other, and where it takes place, is an unsettled question. At the present time the electrophysiological evidence speaks against the conjecture that signals in both systems simply cooperate additively in activating the dendrites of the Purkinje cells. Each climbing fiber seems to excite its Purkinje cell so strongly that an additional excitation in the parallel fiber system could hardly be effectual. It could be, however, that under normal circumstances the excitation in the parallel fiber system reaches the threshold only for a part of the Purkinje cells, so that a massive excitation in the Purkinje cell layer only comes about if the wave of excitation in the parallel fibers reaches a place where many Purkinje cells are already activated by climbing fibers. It may well be that the activity in the Purkinje cell layer is only effective when it reaches a certain local density.

2. On the other hand, a clock can be used as a stopwatch. I turn on the watch at a certain time; after a time that I want to measure, I put a second signal into the watch and read off the distance that the hand has traveled as a measure of the elapsed time. While in the case of the alarm clock I put in a length and receive a time interval as output (for example 8 hours sleep), here I insert a time, and receive as output its transformation into a distance. Applying the idea of the stopwatch to the cerebellar cortex, one could imagine that after the

input of a signal in a particular place in the mossy fiber-parallel fiber system, a question is put so to speak to the cerebellar cortex at a later time by a short, but diffuse excitation of the climbing fiber system. If we assume again that a certain density of excitation in the Purkinje cells can only be reached where climbing fibers and parallel fibers exert excitation at the same time, this will only happen at the place where the excitatory wave in the parallel fiber system has just arrived when the test volley arrives in the climbing fiber system. The distance of this place from the place of input in the parallel fiber system is analogous to the distance through which the hand of the stopwatch has moved, a measure of expired time. The synchronous activation of many climbing fibers that this model requires, is in agreement with the electric coupling of neurons that has been observed in the olivary nucleus.

We can imagine several other applications for a system of delay lines such as evidently exists in the cerebellar cortex. If two signals are fed into the two ends of a delay line, and if they are allowed to interfere locally with each other in a multiplicative fashion, the so-called cross-correlation function can be read off along the line. For instance, if both signals are the same function of time, except that there is a time shift between one and the other, the time-average of the product .will have a maximum at a point corresponding to the time-shift (in the middle for time shift $= 0$, to the right for positive, to the left for negative time shifts). Engineers will have no difficulty appraising the general usefulness of a system of delay lines with provision for multiple tapping along the way.

The basic question, however, is this: what purpose can such space-time and time-space transformations serve in those performances of the nervous system in which the cerebellum apparently is involved, namely, the preservation of equilibrium and the coordination of fine movements? It is not difficult to imagine in what context the measurement of time delays could be important for the coordination of rapid movements. Whoever plays the violin knows how different kinds of bowing can be produced by moving the various joints of the right upper extremity (shoulder, elbow, wrist, finger joints) in different phase-relations to each other. The wrist movement can lag behind that of the elbow, or it may lead, or the two may work synchronously. Conscious concentration on single muscles cannot produce the required delicate differences in the timing of these motions: rather, it disturbs. The movement must be grasped as a whole, and it is then programmed in detail by an unconscious mechanism. The timing of the various phases of complex movements must be very precise and might well be the specialty of the cerebellum. Whether playing musical instruments, throwing stones, or writing fast, milliseconds or tenths of milliseconds are at stake, as can easily be calculated when the speed of motion and the required precision are known. It is interesting to compare this with the accuracy of the cerebellar clock calculated from the speed of signals in the parallel fibers and from the separation of neighboring Purkinje cells. About a tenth of a millisecond is the shortest interval of time that the cerebellar cortex can resolve in the direction of the parallel fibers, which fits in well.

We should discuss the role of the cerebellum proposed here as an alternative to a widely held view of the cerebellum as "the head ganglion of the proprioceptive system," as a kind of central computer in which all information about the present condition of the motor apparatus is united for inclusion in the planning of the next movement. This opinion is apparently based on the observation that when the cerebellum is injured, ataxia sometimes occurs, a particular kind of clumsiness in moving reminiscent of that which accompanies lesions of the spinal cord in which the proprioceptive fibers are destroyed. These are the pathways that normally provide information about the position of the parts of the body relative to each other. The fact that in disturbances of the cerebellar function a particular kind of tremor is often present, which only involves an arm if it carries out a movement directed toward a goal, led Norbert Wiener to his own interpretation of cerebellar function, which he presented in his book *Cybernetics* as a model example of the application of concepts from communication science to the nervous system. The proprioceptive input, together with the movement which follows it, and which in turn produces proprioceptive input, forms a feedback circuit that contiuously maintains the limbs in the desired position. Since it is well known that periodic oscillations belong to the ordinary types of failures in a feedback circuit, Wiener was not at all surprised about the tremor in cerebellar patients. On the contrary, he saw in it a confirmation of the current opinion about the role of the cerebellum in proprioception.

The tables can however be turned. Certainly feedback circuits are involved in standing upright and in slow movements in which signals of the nervous system that generate muscle tension, and those signals that relay information about the generated tension back into the nervous system influence each other. It is also not to be doubted that this feedback circuit will oscillate under certain circumstances, just like other feedback circuits, for example, if it is subjected to a more rapid variation of the input values than it is able to follow, because of the delays involved in the transmission. Therefore, it can be assumed that these feedback circuits are turned off during rapid movements and that such movements are preprogrammed in their entire course. The activation of the single muscles involved takes place without dependence on a reply from the motor organ. The cerebellum is responsible for such rapid movements: if it fails, then the rapid movements must be controlled by means of the proprioceptive feedback circuits. The temporal insufficiency of this mechanism becomes apparent in that oscillations make their appearance − the characteristic "intention tremor" of cerebellar patients.

Less obvious, on first sight, is the role that a millisecond clock plays in the preservation of equilibrium. Yet the cerebellum of all animals is closely tied to the brain centers that receive fibers from the receptors for linear and rotational acceleration in the so-called vestibular nuclei. Lesions of the cerebellum often produce distinct disturbances of equilibrium. In its rudimentary form, in *Cyclostomes,* the cerebellum is nothing more than a bridge of nerve tissue with parallel fibers and Purkinje cells between the right and left vestibular nuclei. In view of this connection to the obviously more static than dynamic function of equilibrium, can the idea of the cerebellum as a timing device still be upheld? I believe that one can show that in swimming aquatic animals (which prehistoric vertebrates that first developed a cerebellum certainly were) the problem of stabilization against rotation around a longitudinal axis could be best solved by a mechanism involving temporal coding.

A cross section of an idealized cylindrical fish is represented in Figure 6.3. Dorsal fin and anal fin are drawn as two pointers that mark the up–down direction of the fish. We imagine that all corrections of deviations from the normal, vertical position are achieved through the movement of 2 lateral fins (pectoral fins). Each of the fins beats downward, whereby the left one produces a clockwise rotation of the fish and the right one, a counterclockwise rotation. From the many possible ways of controlling this correcting mechanism, I will pick out two extremes, one, so to speak, with cerebellum, the other without.

First, without the cerebellum: the fish perceives a deviation by an angle α from his normal position, either by means of his sense of equilibrium, or because he sees the horizon slanted. He reacts with his right fin with which he gives his body a rotational acceleration precisely calculated so that, when the vertical position is reached, the frictional force that works against the rotation will have just annulled it. If the normal position is not reached, or if the correction overshoots the mark, a second fin stroke, either right or left, can bring

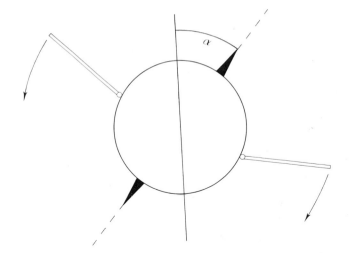

FIGURE 6.3. Correction of a deviation from the upright position by means of two pectoral fins. Explanation in the text

about a further correction, etc., until the desired position is reached. The magnitude of the deviation in this scheme is translated into the magnitude of the correcting force. The force that is used has to be quite small if it is to be counterbalanced by friction in water, therefore the correction is slow. Precision is unsatisfactory, since all kinds of disturbances that may be caused by movements in the surrounding water are relatively strong compared to the corrective forces.

The second model is with the cerebellum. The correction happens by means of a forceful fin stroke of always the same strength and duration. The angular momentum imparted to the fish is annulled, when a position of equilibrium is reached, by an equally large angular momentum of opposite sign produced by a fin stroke on the other side. The forces in question are large compared to the frictional force and to random disturbances. Therefore the correction comes about rapidly and can be precisely calculated. The measure of the deviation from the normal position is translated into the time interval between the fin stroke on one side and that on the other. The decisive advantage is that the correction by two opposite, equally large, but time-shifted pulses always leaves the fish motionless after the completed correction, no matter if the correction has been perfect, or imprecise. I propose the conjecture that the cerebellum first developed as an organ specialized for space–time transformations in connection with the regulation of the vertical position by means of pairs of phase-shifted symmetric movements.

If we wanted to go beyond these general observations, it would not be difficult to invent some more fairly plausible schemes involving the translation of positional information into positive and negative delays (and vice versa). The independent motion of our arms and legs on the background of their coordinated interplay in the maintainance of equilibrium offers ample opportunity for creative speculation. I will not elaborate further on this since that would lead us far away from that which, at the present time, can be experimentally upheld. Whether or not temporal aspects are involved in the coordination of movement and, particularly, in the preservation of a stable position in space is a question that calls for experimentation. For the present, it is enough for us to have brought up conjectures based on the observation of structure. The proof demands a technique foreign to the anatomist. Even brain science will, unfortunately, not be able to escape specialization.

A general consideration is still appropriate for those who feel at home in the theory of scientific method. The thought that the task of the cerebellum is to measure time can be used as an hypothesis which should be tested experimentally, as is right and proper for all hypotheses. In the attempt to set this into practice, one encounters a difficulty of principle, however. One can experimentally prove, for example, that signals in the parallel fiber system arrive at different times at different Purkinje cells in a row, as Freeman [6.6] showed with electrophysiologic technique. What is proved, however, is merely what one has read out of the structure anyway, something that simply emerges from the known facts of the limited speed of conduction in nerve fibers and of the synaptic connections between neurons. Whether the production of intervals of time is actually the purpose of the cerebellar structure, as the hypothesis reads, or whether the delays are merely an unplanned side effect, is a question that cannot be answered experimentally. Explanations involving purpose, teleologic interpretations, illuminate facts in a way similar to causal explanations, but one must be aware that, in principle, only those cases can be verified in which the engineer who built the thing can be asked what his intentions had been. This can certainly not be done with brains.

References

6.1   Braitenberg, V.: Is the cerebellar cortex a biological clock in the millisecond range? In: Progress in Brain Research. The Cerebellum. Amsterdam: Elsevier 25, 334–346 (1967)

6.2   Braitenberg, V., Atwood, R.P.: Morphological observations on the cerebellar cortex. J. Comp. Neurol. *109*, 1–34 (1958)

6.3   Braitenberg, V., Onesto, N.: The cerebellar cortex as a timing organ. Discussion of a hypothesis. Proc. 1st Intern. Conf. Medical Cybernetics, Naples. 3–19 (1960)

6.4   Dow, R.S., Moruzzi, G.: The Physiology and Pathology of the Cerebellum. Univ. Minneapolis: Minnesota Press, 1958

6.5   Eccles, J.C., Ito, M., Szentágothai, J.: The Cerebellum as a Neuronal Machine. Berlin-Heidelberg-New York: Springer 1967

6.6   Freeman, J.A.: The cerebellum as a timing device. An experimental study in the frog. In: Neurobiology of Cerebellar Evolution and Development. Chicago: Am. Med. Assoc. Llinas (ed.) 1969, p. 397

6.7   Griesinger, W.: Die Pathologie und Therapie der psychischen Krankheiten. Stuttgart: Adolph Krabbe, 1861

6.8   Llinas, R. (ed.): Neurobiology of Cerebellar Evolution and Development. Chicago: Am. Med. Assoc., 1969

6.9   Llinas, R., Baker, R., Sotelo, C.: Electrotonic coupling between neurons in cat inferior olive. J. Neurophysiol. *37*, 560–571 (1974)

6.10 Nicholson, C., Llinas, R., Precht, W.: Neural elements of the cerebellum in elasmobranch fishes: Structural and functional characteristics. In: Llinas (ed.) Neurobiology of Cerebellar Evolution and Development. Chicago: Am. Med. Assoc. 1969, p. 215

6.11 Sotelo, C., Llinas, R., Baker, R.: Structural study of inferior olivary nucleus of the cat: Morphological correlates of electrotonic coupling. J. Neurophysiol. *37*, 541–559 (1974)

6.12 Weyl, H.: Symmetry. Princeton Univ. Press, 1952

7. The Automatic Pilot of the Fly

> *It has always seemed to me extreme presumptuousness on the part of those who want to make human ability the measure of what nature can and knows how to do, since, when one comes down to it, there is not one effect in nature, no matter how small, that even the most speculative minds can fully understand.*   *Galileo Galilei [7.4]*

An extreme view of the relation between psychology and brain anatomy, a view I would not have dared to advance if the subject of this Chapter had been humans rather than flies, is the following: a thorough analysis of behavior must result in a scheme that shows all regularities that are to be found between the sensory input and the motor output of the animal. This scheme is an abstract representation of the brain. If we are lucky, its structure can be identified with the structure of the fiber patterns within the brain that constitute the mechanism tested in the behavioral experiments. If we are not so lucky, the structure of the behavioral scheme may not be the same as that of the brain, but may still be equivalent to it, in the sense that both belong to a class of structures that perform the same function and therefore cannot be distinguished in the behavioral experiment. From this point of view, psychology (analysis of behavior) is a source of hypotheses on brain structure, a subsidiary branch of brain anatomy. Conversely, anatomy could be understood as a method of psychology, as the most direct means of understanding the structural complexity that constitutes the mind.

I would now like to show how, in the relatively simple system of visually guided navigation in flies, the discussion on structure occurs at a level in which the comparison of fibers in the brain with elements of behavior clearly goes beyond abstract speculation. We mentioned the visual ganglia of the fly in connection with the precision of fiber patterns in nerve nets (Chap. 5). Now we will consider them from another point of view: as mechanisms in which signals from the eyes are analyzed and transformed in order to contribute intelligently to the behavior of the animal.

When we say "to see" we think first of seeing shapes. This is perhaps because for us humans, the most important function of the visual mechanism is to pick out forms from the surrounding space in order to compare them to the forms stored in memory, in other words, to identify and recognize the objects in our environment. It could also be the result of an ancient philosophical outlook, whereby the essential elements of thought are the "forms" of objects, (original meaning: molds or impressions) and in particular the impressions of visually perceived objects, "the ideas", a word that derives from the Greek word for vision.

Everyone who has not sacrificed his observational powers to the traditional abstractions of philosophers has noticed that in reality we do not see the rigid forms of things, but almost always forms in motion, forms around which we move, or forms that we scan with our eye movements.

This seeing of movements, and not of rigid outlines, certainly plays the main part in the fly's eye. The very poor angular resolution of the compound eye is sufficient evidence for this. Two points of light cannot be identified as separate by the fly if they are not more than 2° from each other. Even in the peripheral regions of the human eye, whose reduced visual ability one can easily test by fixating a point and attempting to describe how much one sees of objects that are distant from it, the resolution is still quite a bit better than that of the fly. What does the fly see with its imposing compound eyes apparently so little suited for recognizing objects?

Without doubt the answer is: it sees mainly movements, the flowing past of the visual surroundings when it flies, the apparent rotation of the panorama when it turns in one place, the passing by of single details which it comes close to, certainly also the movements of other animals in its environment, and much else.

One can easily imagine in which situations this might be important, and it is an interesting game to think up mechanisms, of vital importance for the animal, that would detect particularly significant distributions of movements in the visual field of the fly and release the appropriate motor reactions. For example:

Figure 7.1 shows a fly from above flying down a long corridor. The visual field, actually a horizontal section through it, is drawn around the fly with arrows drawn in at different places, whose length and direction represent the speed and direction of the perceived movement. At the very front and back the perceived movement is 0; at the sides, at right angles to the direction of flight, the speed is greatest, in fact the greater, the narrower the corridor. In addition to this

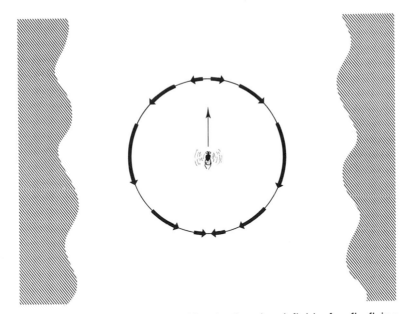

FIGURE 7.1. Distribution of velocities in the visual field of a fly flying through a narrow corridor

information about the distance of the walls, the fly can learn much more about its environment from the distribution of the motion in its visual field. If the 0-point lies somewhere at the side and not at the front, this means that the fly is being driven sideways from its direction of flight, for example by a current of air. If the point lies above or below and not horizontally to the front, the fly can conclude that it is diverted either above or below its line of flight. A set of movement detectors aptly distributed over the visual field can be used to trigger the maneuvers that will correct these deviations.

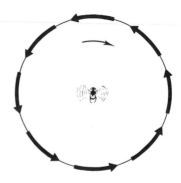

FIGURE 7.2. Distribution of velocities in the visual field of a fly turning around a vertical axis

Figure 7.2 shows another and certainly very important situation. The fly rotates around a vertical axis and therefore sees a movement in the opposite direction having the same angular velocity in the whole field. From this it can compute the changes in its position with respect to the coordinates of the environment. If it wants to return to the original position, it has to rotate in the direction of the apparent movement that it has seen. If the fly possessed a mechanism that could translate a rotational movement of the visual field into an activation of the motor system so that after a change in its course it would tend to come back to the original direction, it would be well stabilized against chance deviations in forward flight.

Moreover, one can visualize the environment of the fly as consisting of separate objects situated at various distances. A small object on a uniform or distant background (Fig. 7.3) will generate a percep-

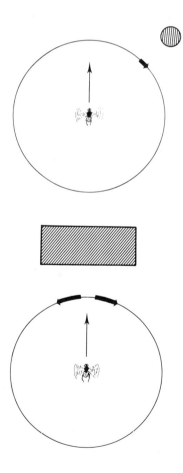

FIGURE 7.3. Distribution of velocities in the visual field of a fly flying past a small object in front of a structureless background

FIGURE 7.4. Distribution of velocities in the visual field of a fly approaching a landing surface

tion of movement in a circumscribed area of the visual field when the fly flies past it. This small spot of visual movement could signify to the fly an island of salvation in the three-dimensional ocean of air in which it moves, and one would be happy to equip the insect with a mechanism for discovering such exceptional regions in the environment in order to guide the flight to a landing there.

If the fly flies straight toward an object that rises out of the environment directly in front of it (Fig. 7.4), it sees a pattern of divergent movement in front, an ever faster streaming motion in all directions. It would be sensible to use this particular perception as the trigger to a mechanism that governs the complicated, but stereotyped landing maneuvers of the fly.

Our speculation as to what kinds of perceptions of movement could be useful for the fly does not seem to be far off the mark, since it leads to results that match the physiological mechanisms that evidently proved useful in evolution. The various distributions of movement in the visual field in the situations illustrated in Figures 7.1 to 7.4 can also be artificially created in the laboratory in order to test the

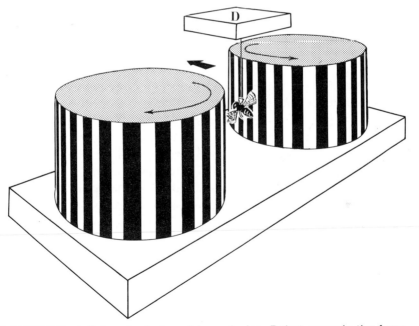

FIGURE 7.5. A flying fly fastened to a device D that records the force developed in the direction of flight. The two rotating cylinders simulate a panorama of stripes moving backward. The angle between the long axis of the fly and that of the cylinders can be varied

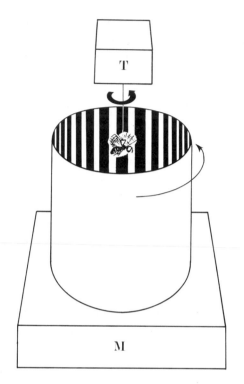

FIGURE 7.6. A flying fly fastened to a device *T* that records the torque exerted around a vertical axis. The fly is surrounded by a hollow cylinder painted with black and white stripes inside and driven by a motor *M*

fly's reactions (Figs. 7.5, 7.6). In each case the fly reacts in a way that suggests appropriate purposeful behavior. The movement that flows by on both sides in the same direction (Fig. 7.1) influences the force developed in the forward direction of flight, or in other words, the speed of flight and therefore, indirectly, the altitude of flight (Fig. 7.5). The rotation of a panorama in the visual field of the fly (Fig. 7.2), which can easily be simulated by a cylinder rotating around the fly, is given the appropriate response: the fly turns in the same direction as the cylinder, as if it knew that this type of rotation of the visual field normally occurs as a consequence of its own deviation in the opposite direction (Fig. 7.6). If a fly flying around is shown a marking on a structureless background, such as a branch on the background of the sky, it turns toward it. This reaction is generated by the to- and fro motion of the image of the object in a small area of the visual field (which, in turn, is a consequence of the fly's own wiggling motion). If the fly is offered a divergent, streaming motion originating from a point in the forward part of the visual field (Fig. 7.4), for example, by turning a disc on which a spiral is drawn, one can observe how the fly prepares to land by stretching out its legs, which are otherwise tucked close to the body during flight.

These experiments[9] give a convincing picture of the characteristics of motion perception in insects. I will summarize the most important points as far as they apply to flies. Then we should try to relate the structure of the visual ganglia to the results of behavioral analysis.

1. Movement is perceived on the basis of a computation of the inputs to two neighboring channels, as a result, so to speak, of the comparison of that which neighboring "visual rays" see.

This statement is not as obvious as it may seem. A rudimentary type of detection of movement could, for example, take place in a single channel in which the flicker frequency, perceived in the single channel, is used as a measure of the speed of a moving striped pattern. A condition for this is that the spacing of the stripes in the pattern be known: a snapshot produced by many channels in parallel could give information on this. It could also have been that not just two, but many channels were necessary for each elementary perception of movement, in the case that movement in the visual field triggered a physiological event only when a long row of receptors were activated in succession. Or, possibly, the brain could detect movement in the visual field by comparing the inputs of two visual channels lying far apart from each other. None of these alternatives seems to be the case, or better, if other mechanisms for perception of movement exist, these seem to play a less important role than that which involves the comparison of inputs of two neighboring channels.

This is known from an experiment that can be understood in its essentials by studying Figure 7.7. A periodic pattern, the chain of black pearls to the right in the picture (we must imagine the chain extended at both ends), is drawn past a row of receptors R_1, R_2, and R_3. When a pearl passes a receptor it is "seen" by it. What each receptor sees over a certain period of time, is indicated by the black dots on the three lines; the image of each pearl runs obliquely over this space–time diagram (dashed lines). Imagine a movement detector that functions according to the principle that a receptor that sees a particular event, asks the neighboring receptors if one of them has seen the same event shortly before. An affirmative answer by one of the two neighboring receptors can be taken as indication of a movement that has taken place in the corresponding direction. Look at the event at the present time t_0 on the receptor R_2 at A. Questioning the

---

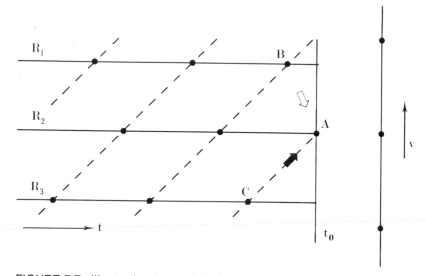

FIGURE 7.7. Illustration to explain the apparent movement in the opposite direction that is perceived when a moving periodic pattern is seen by a periodic array of receptors whose spacing is slightly less than the period of the pattern. The moving pattern is supposed to be a string of pearls moving with the velocity *v*. The distance between successive pearls is $\frac{3}{2}$ that between the receptors R1 and R2, R2 and R3. The dotted oblique lines crossing the space–time plot on the left side of the picture represent the trajectories of the images of successive pearls. The comparison of the time at which neighboring receptors perceive a pearl could lead to the supposition of a movement (*white arrow at A*) in a direction opposite to that of the real movement *(black arrow)*. t_0: present time

neighboring receptors results in the answer that a similar event was seen shortly before by R_1 (B). From this we might erroneously construe a movement from R_1 to R_2 (white arrow) that seems even more rapid than the movement that actually took place from R_3 to R_2 (black arrow from C to A). Altogether, on the basis of the sum of the true and the false movements, this motor receptor would indicate movement in the direction opposite to that which has really occurred. Such illusions can be expected if the wavelength of the pattern in motion (in this case, the distance between the pearls) is smaller than twice the distance between the receptors. Indeed, if striped patterns are moved within the visual field of a fly, and the stripes are made increasingly narrower, a point is reached at which the reaction of the fly to the movement results in moving in the opposite, instead of in the same direction. We may conclude from this that the fly now sees

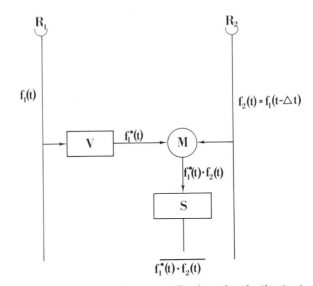

FIGURE 7.8. A movement detector. Explanation in the text

the movement in the opposite direction, in accordance with the explanation of Figure 7.7. From the wavelength of the pattern, at which the reaction just changes from the normal to the opposite direction, we can calculate the angular separation between receptors involved in movement detection. The result coincides with the measured angle between the visual axes of neighboring ommatidia of the fly's eye. This leads us to our statement that perception of motion takes place between neighboring channels of the compound eye.

2. The mechanisms that discover movement between neighboring channels, in short: the movement detectors are distributed throughout the entire visual field.

This is known from the following experiment [7.5]. A fly flying inside a rotating striped cylinder is fastened to an apparatus that measures the rotational tendency (i.e., the torque) with which it answers the perceived movement. The fly does not see the whole cylinder, but merely that part that it can see through a window in a screen placed between it and the cylinder. The reaction of the fly becomes greater, the larger the window is made. If the window is made higher, then more motion detectors are stimulated in parallel. If it is made wider, each stripe of the cylinder stimulates more movement detectors one after the other. Both cases lead to an increase of the reaction of the fly, and prove to us that movement detectors all over the visual field contribute to the perception of movement.

3. The central part of each movement detector in the fly is an element by which signals from neighboring channels are multiplied with each other.

This concept, developed by Hassenstein and Reichardt in an analysis of movement detection in another insect, the beetle *Chlorophanus,* is true also of the fly.

More exactly, the movement detector (Fig. 7.8) consists of a short-term memory that delays signals from one channel with respect to those from the other channel, of a multiplier, and of a mechanism that calculates the time average of the multiplier output. These three parts of the movement detectors correspond to very simple electronic devices. Together they form not a perfect, but still a useful mechanism for the discovery of movement between two receptors. This can be understood as follows:

First the multiplier: I can use it to discover how similar two processes of time are, $f_1(t)$ and $f_2(t)$, which, for simplicity's sake, I will assume are not periodic, are symmetrically distributed about zero [the temporal average of $f_1(t)$ and of $f_2(t)$ is equal to zero], and take on the same values with equal frequency. If I continually multiply $f_1(t)$ with $f_2(t)$ and let the result of this product add up in a memory store for a certain length of time, I receive the highest value in the memory if $f_1(t)$ is identical with $f_2(t)$. One need only consider then that all values of the product are always positive, since positive values of $f_1(t)$ are always multiplied with positive values of $f_2(t)$, negative values with negative values. If both processes of time are not identical, the less "similar" they are, the more the positive values of $f_1(t)$ will be multiplied with negative values of $f_2(t)$ or the other way around, whereby the product takes on negative values each time. If both processes are totally dissimilar, if they have nothing to do with each other, it will occur exactly as often that both values have the same sign at the same time as that they have opposite signs, which results in the values of the products being as often positive as negative, and zero in the temporal average.

The box, V, in Figure 7.8 functions as a short-term memory in that it does not immediately pass on signals that reach it, but drags them out in time, so to speak. An illustration of the action of such a mechanism can be seen in Figure 7.9. What the single receptor sees is a series of white and black stripes on a uniformly gray background [$f_1(t)$ in Fig. 7.9]. After having passed through the short-term memory, each stripe of the original series turns into a slowly diminishing signal, which is illustrated by the smudging of the stripe on the record labeled $f_1^*(t)$ in Figure 7.9. This corresponds to the effect of certain

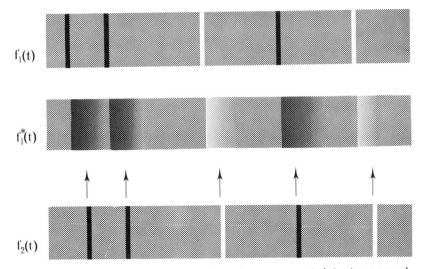

FIGURE 7.9. Explanation of the action of a movement detector according to the Hassenstein–Reichardt model. The time course of the input to two neighboring visual channels of the compound eye is represented as the succession of gray, black, and white in the two bands $f_1(t)$ and $f_2(t)$, respectively. The horizontal coordinate in these plots represents time. If the two inputs are produced by a pattern of stripes moving by the visual receptors, $f_2(t)$ will be equal to $f_1(t)$, only shifted by a certain amount depending on the velocity (the smaller, the greater the velocity). The "short-term memory" V of Figure 7.8 transforms the input $f_1(t)$ into the sequence of smudged signals $f_1^*(t)$, which is then compared to the input $f_2(t)$ (*arrows*). The product $f_1^*(t) \cdot f_2(t)$, averaged over time, is the greater, the smaller the time shift between $f_1(t)$ and $f_2(t)$, i.e., the greater the velocity of the moving pattern

filters, made from a condenser and a resistor, upon a pulse of electric current in an electronic circuit, or to the effect of an elastic rubber hose on shocks of water pressure, or to the effect of a heavy tile stove on the daily charges of heat.

The combined action of multiplier and short-term memory now becomes understandable (Fig. 7.8). If the multiplier is used to determine the similarity between two temporal processes, I can now, on the one hand, feed it the input of receptor R_1 transformed by V, and on the other, the input of receptor R_2 directly, and will find the more "similarity", the less of a time shift Δt there is between the process $f_2(t)$ in receptor R_2 and $f_1(t)$ in R_1. Remember that the whole arrangement is supposed to discover the movement of a panorama, here schematically represented by a series of white and black stripes on gray. Both receptors see the same temporal sequence of events but not at

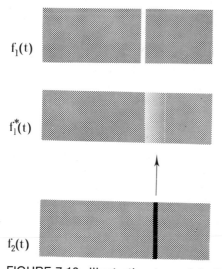

FIGURE 7.10. Illustration to explain the optomotor reaction in the direction opposite to the direction of a moving pattern that one obtains when the stripes change from white to black (or vice versa) on their way from one receptor to the next. In this case, the product $f_1(t)^* \cdot f_2(t)$ is always negative. Such experiments show that the basic operation of the movement detector must be something akin to multiplication

the same time. The difference in time is the smaller, the higher the velocity with which the panorama moves. Comparing the sequence $f_2(t)$ with the smudged sequence $f_1^*(t)$, each black (white) stripe in $f_2(t)$ corresponds to a point in $f_1^*(t)$ that is the blacker (the whiter), the faster the movement. The average of the product $f_1^*(t) \cdot f_2(t)$ will have a value that increases with increasing velocity. The memory S contains, after a certain time, a measure of the speed of a pattern moving past a receptor.

It could be that in reality things are somewhat more complicated than I have presented them here, since I have purposely withheld several difficulties. Those who would like more information on the development of this model of the perception of movement, based originally on a beetle, should read References [7.7, 7.13, and 7.14]. The application to flies and the further development of this research in many rich ramifications can be read in References [7.3, 7.5, 7.6, 7.9, 7.10, and 7.12].

Just one further remark on the kind of experiment that has led to the assumption of a multiplicative interaction as a basis of the perception of movement between two receptors. Figure 7.10 shows an experiment, schematically simplified, in which the animal is offered a series of input signals that normally do not occur. One receptor, R_1, sees a white stripe, and the other one, R_2, sees a black one shortly thereafter. The moving object has changed its appearance, so to speak, on the way. The reaction of the animal is correspondingly paradox: it reacts as if it had seen movement in the opposite direction. This can be interpreted as a result of the multiplication of the signals between the two channels. Normally the two channels see the same signals one after the other: one "light" and then the other "light," or one "dark" and then the other "dark." If one takes "light" as a positive signal, "dark" as a negative one, the product in both cases of either two positive or two negative magnitudes will be positive. If positive follows negative, or vice versa, the negative values will be multiplied with positive values: the result has a negative sign.

4. The next assertion is already implicitly included in the description of a movement detector as we have just sketched it, but it is worthwhile to point it out separately.

Movement detectors are oriented. They discriminate between movements in opposite directions. Not only the magnitude, but also the direction of the velocity vector is seen. Of course, what counts is the projection of a movement in the visual field onto a line connecting the two input points; in other words, the length of the velocity vector times the cosine of the angle between its direction, and the direction in which the movement detector is situated between two receptors. A movement perpendicular to this is not seen.

5. Where movement can be seen in a particular direction (for example from front to rear), there it can also be seen in the opposite direction (for example from the rear to the front.)

This can be interpreted in different ways. Either there is only one movement detector between every two receptors, which is excited by movement in either direction and which can distinguish between the two (by emitting positive signals for one direction and negative ones for the other), or there are two movement detectors between every two receptors, one for each direction. The question as to which of the two schemes is actually realized is still open.

6. The movement detectors cannot all have the same orientation, for example, they cannot all be arranged either horizontally or vertically. There must be at least 2 sets of them oriented in two different directions, because there are experimental situations in which vertical movement in the visual field is maximally effective, horizontal movement not at all, and other experimental situations in which the opposite is true. This is not compatible with a common orientation of all movement detectors.

This is known from a series of experiments by Götz on the fruitfly *Drosophila* (later also confirmed on the housefly). Movement streaming by on both sides of the animal in the same direction, such as a fly would see it when it flies a straight course, in turn influences the velocity of flight. This depends, however, on the direction. If the panorama in the visual field moves upward on both sides, the velocity of flight increases; if it moves downward, it decreases. Only if the streaming occurs horizontally, from the front to the rear, or from the rear to the front, does the velocity remain unchanged (Fig. 7.5). The movement detectors whose excitation is transferred into the control of the velocity of flight (in *Drosophila* simply into the amplitude of the wing beat, and consequently, into the thrust in a forward and upward direction) seem to be inserted between two neighboring channels along the vertical direction of the eye. This is quite different in the preceding experiments in which the panorama (e. g., a cylinder with stripes painted inside) turns around the fly (Fig. 7.6) and in which the fly reacts with a deviation from straight flight; i. e., with an asymmetry of the forces produced by the right and left wings. Here, too, the direction (on both sides in opposite directions) of the streaming movement can be changed by tilting the axis of rotation of the cylinder, and reactions of varying strengths will be observed. The tendency to turn in the same direction as the cylinder is strongest in the fly when the cylinder turns around a vertical axis, and the panorama streams past toward the front on one side, toward the rear on the other, whereas the rotation of the cylinder around a horizontal axis (the panorma streaming upward on one side, downward on the other) causes no asymmetry of the force developed on both sides during flight. In this case the movement detectors involved seem to be inserted between two neighboring channels in the horizontal direction, in contrast to the foregoing experiment.

At this juncture it should be said that by just looking at the behavior we cannot distinguish between one system in which the movement detectors are actually oriented in a horizontal and a vertical direction, and one in which they lie between the receptors in two other (oblique) directions, since the vertical and horizontal movement in the visual field could be computed from their projections onto any two nonparallel coordinates. We only know for sure that the movement detectors must be oriented in at least two directions, since if they all had the same orientation, they could not distinguish between movements in two different directions that were symmetric to the orientation of the movement detector.

Whoever has read to here may perhaps ask why I present a fascinating chapter of exact behavioral research in such detail, when

I started out by making propaganda for a different science, that of neuroanatomy. The two branches of research are methodically almost opposed: on the one hand, behavioral research with its ambition to understand the structures underlying behavior without opening the container in which responsible mechanisms lie, and on the other hand, anatomy with the assertion that behavior of the living being can be read off the structure of fiber connections in the dead animal. Actually a dialogue between two partners trying to uncover the same situation by looking at it from opposite ends is here certainly the most sensible course. What we anatomists gain from such a dialogue is at least this: the laws of the distribution, position, and orientation of movement detectors, as we extract them from the results of behavioral research, can easily be converted to a want ad for fibers that we can actually look for in the structure of the visual ganglia.

Such a want ad, a hypothesis for neuroanatomical use that we can extract from behavioral experiments about movement perception may read as follows:

We are looking for fibers that connect neighboring channels in the visual ganglia of the fly with each other. There must be at least two systems of such fibers, arranged in two different directions, either vertical and horizontal, or in other directions that are probably symmetric with respect to the horizontal direction. Each fiber has different connections with both channels between which it relays signals. These fibers form a continuous net spread over the whole ganglion.

The description of these fibers is a consequence of what one knows about the movement detectors (propositions 1–6 above) and of the assumption that signal transmission within the mechanism for movement detection occurs via nerve fibers. That these fibers are to be looked for somewhere in the three visual ganglia, and not somewhere else in the nervous system of the fly, follows from the fact that electrophyiologists [7.1, 7.8] have recorded signals from single neurons at the end of the chain of the visual ganglia, which could only be elicited by a movement in the visual field. The detection of a movement on the basis of a comparison of the input from neighboring receptors must have already occurred between the point where the microelectrode was, and the periphery of the visual system.

Are there such fibers in the brain of the fly? Very soon I shall probably be able to give a more precise answer to this question, which is at present of central interest to fly neuroanatomists. So much can already be said: There are fibers in at least two levels of the chain of visual ganglia that connect neighboring channels in the two oblique directions of the hexagonal array which is recognizable everywhere in the visual ganglia, and which mirrors the tesselation of the visual field by means of the 2 times 3000 visual rays. If individual ommatidia correspond to single lines of sight, one can assume that a fiber connecting two neighboring ommatidia is used for the computation of the two inputs from the corresponding lines of sight.

A fiber system like this, right below the first visual ganglion, is illustrated in Figures 5.7 and 5.8 and has already been discussed in connection with the question of the precision of wiring. From each fiber bundle (each position of the array of ommatidia) a fiber sends out a branch to the neighboring fiber bundles above and to the rear, and below and to the rear. There the terminations of these branches, as can easily be seen in the electron microscope, make a true synaptic connection with other fibers of the neighboring bundles – and with each other (Chapter 5). More than this can hardly be said about the function of these small fibers at the present time. They are, however, not the best candidates for the role in movement perception, as we have defined it in our want ad. One of the reasons for this is that it is difficult to reconcile the reciprocal synapses that these fibers have with each other with the logical structure of a set of movement detectors.

The fibers most likely indicted by circumstantial evidence are located at a different level, near the surface of the second visual ganglion, the medulla. They run in two oblique directions between the levels of the medulla at which various kinds of fibers from the first visual ganglion, the lamina ganglionaris, terminate. Two of these lamina-medulla relay neurons, L_1 and L_2 in our terminology, are particularly interesting, since in each compartment (neuro-ommatidium or cartridge) of the lamina they seem to receive exactly the same information from the corresponding line of sight, judging from their identical synaptic contacts with the primary afferent fibers. The shape of their bodies and, especially, the shape and position of their terminal knobs in the medulla are, however, very different: it is very tempting to interpret them as the two inputs to the multiplier that forms the heart of each movement detector. The two input lines must have different properties (electronically speaking they must contain different filters) in order to give the movement detector the asymmetry that is required if it is to distinguish between movements in the two opposite directions. If L_1 and L_2 are the filters, then the neurons that are interposed between the termination of L_1 in one channel and that of L_2 in the neighboring channel might well be the multipliers. Farther down, possibly in the third visual ganglion (the lobula complex), we might look for the integrators, separate for each direction, which compute the time averages (Fig. 7.11, cf. also Fig. 7.8).

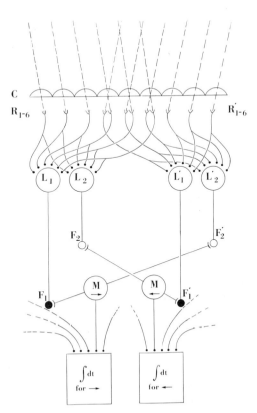

FIGURE 7.11. Illustration of a hypothesis on the position of the movement detectors in the visual system of the fly. The upper part of the
diagram is a crude summary of the situation illustrated in Figure 5.3.
Two sets of visual receptors, R_{1-6} and R'_{1-6}, sharing in part the lenses of
the compound eye C, receive visual input from two different directions
in the visual field (*dotted lines*). Each set makes synaptic connections of
exactly the same sort with a pair of neurons in the lamina ganglionaris,
L_1, L_2 and L_1', L_2', respectively. The different shapes of these neurons
makes it likely that L_1 and L_2 transform the identical input in different
ways. Their terminations, symbolized by the black and white disks F_1
and F_2 (F_1' and F_2', respectively) are at different levels of the second
visual ganglion, the medulla. One may interpret L_1 and L_2 as the different filters interposed between the two receptors and the multiplier in the
Reichardt-Hassenstein model (simplified in Fig. 7.8, V). They are required to make the movement detector asymmetric and thus, directional. The element that performs the multiplication (*M*) would then be
housed in the layer of the medulla between that of the terminations F_1
and F_2. There would be two such elements between two input channels,
one for each direction of movement. The integration of the output of all
multiplying units might occur at the level of the third visual ganglion,
the lobula complex, which contains very large neurons (boxes at the
bottom of the diagram)

Of course, the proof or disproof of these identifications of histologic elements with entities postulated on the basis of behavioral experiments will come from direct electrophysiologic evidence. At present, the refined techniques of insect electrophysiologists have almost, but not quite, reached the spatial resolution necessary for a systematic characterization of all the neurons involved.

References

7.1   Bishop, L. G., Keehn, D. G.: Two types of motion sensitive neurons in the optic lobe of the fly. Nature (London) *212*, 1374–1376 (1966)
7.2   Braitenberg, V., Taddei Ferretti, C.: Landing reaction of *musca domestica* induced by visual stimuli. Naturwissenschaften *53*, 155 (1966)
7.3   Fermi, G., Reichardt, W.: Optomotorische Reaktion der Fliege Musca domestica. Abhängigkeit der Reaktion von der Wellenlänge, der Geschwindigkeit, dem Kontrast und der mittleren Leuchtdichte bewegter periodischer Muster. Kybernetik *2*, 15–28 (1963)
7.4   Galilei, G.: Dialogo sopra i due massimi sistemi del mondo. Torino: Einaudi Editore, 1970 (Florence 1632)
7.5   Götz, K. G.: Optomotorische Untersuchung des visuellen Systems einiger Augenmutanten der Fruchtfliege *Drosophila*. Kybernetik *2*, 77–92 (1964)
7.6   Götz, K. G.: Flight control in *Drosophila* by visual perception of motion. Kybernetik *2*, 199–208 (1968)
7.7   Hassenstein, B.: Über die Wahrnehmung der Bewegung von Figuren und unregelmäßigen Helligkeitsmustern. Z. vergl. Physiol. *40*, 556–592 (1958)
7.8   Hausen, K.: Functional characterization and anatomical identification of motion sensitive neurons in the lobula plate of the blowfly *Calliphora erythrocephala*. Z. Naturforsch. *31*, 629–633 (1976)
7.9   Kirschfeld, K.: Die Projektion der optischen Umwelt auf das Raster der Rhabdomere im Komplexauge von Musca. Exptl. Brain Res. *3*, 248–270 (1967)
7.10 McCann, G. D., MacGinitie, G. F.: Optomotor response studies of insect vision. Proc. Roy. Soc. Lond. Ser. B *163*, 369–401 (1965)
7.11 Reichardt, W.: The Insect Eye as a Model for Analysis of Uptake, Transduction and Processing of Optical Data in the Nervous System. 34. Physikertagung Salzburg. Stuttgart: Teubner, 1970, pp. 314–353
7.12 Reichardt, W., Poggio, T.: Visual control of orientation behaviour in the fly. Part I. A quantitative analysis Quart. Rev. Biophysics *9*, 311–375 (1976)
7.13 Reichardt, W., Varjú, D.: Übertragungseigenschaften im Auswertesystem für das Bewegungssehen. Z. Naturforsch. *14b* (10), 674–689 (1959)
7.14 Varjú, D., Reichardt, W.: Übertragungseigenschaften im Auswertesystem für das Bewegungssehen II. Z. Naturforsch. *22b* (12), 1343–1351 (1967)

8. The Common Sensorium: An Essay on the Cerebral Cortex*

> *Truth is of two kinds, consisting either in the discovery of the proportions of ideas, considered as such, or in the conformity of our ideas of objects to their real existence.* David Hume [8.13]

> *For the same things can be thought as can be.* Parmenides [8.17]

There is a curious ambiguity in the neuroanatomist's attitude toward the cerebral cortex, the most respected and at the same time the most neglected piece of the human brain. We have learned from the localizationists that the cerebral cortex is responsible for the highest psychic functions, but we do not know what to make of this in view of the stupendous cerebral cortex of a cow, which most nonspecialists can hardly distinguish from that of man. We have also learned that on the surface of the cerebral cortex innumerable "areas" can be distinguished, each devoted to a very special function, but generations of experimental psychologists have piled up evidence to the effect that it does not matter which part of the cortex of a rat is ablated, – the behavior of the animal in their hands is reduced to a degree that depends on the amount, not on the localization of, the tissue destroyed. Some say that the structure of the cerebral cortex is complex beyond description, too complex ever to be understood by the human mind, which, after all, possesses no more complex instrument that the cortex itself to perform the analysis. Others approach the physiology of the cerebral cortex with the same strategy that has been useful in the study of the frog's eye, only to discover that the cortex of the monkey is somewhat simpler than the retina of the frog.

My own approach [8.3–8.5] is similar to that outlined in the Chapter on the cerebellum. We will look for the most general description of the cortical structure, abstracting from the local (i.e., within one brain) and interspecific variations. This approach will be used as a basis for some speculations about the particular sort of data processing for which the cerebral cortex is responsible. The speculation will

---

* To Larry, with thanks.

in turn illuminate various aspects of the cortical anatomy and, in particular, will allow us to make some sense out of various quantitative statements (number of neurons, length of the fibers, etc.).

1. The cerebral cortex is *the largest piece of gray matter* of the mammalian brain (Fig. 8.1). In fact there are two separate cortices, each weighing, in man, about 250 g and thus together occupying about half of the supratentorial cavity, i.e., the portion of the skull above the cerebellum. I think an argument from the sheer size of the cerebral cortex is the strongest point in favor of the view that the cerebral cortex functions, at least in man and his fellow monkeys, as a sort of director general of the brain. We have already briefly discussed (Chaps. 4 and 6) the implications of the continuity of the synaptic web within one piece of gray matter, as opposed to the situation in which different pieces of gray matter are connected together by masses of fibers in the white substance. The absence of well-defined boundaries within the gray substance, the fact that every small region of gray substance contains pieces of dendrites and axons belonging to neurons of the same gray substance, situated at distances that may be very large compared to the macroscopic dimensions of the whole organ, suggests that such an organ functions as a whole. There are no channels within the gray substance that are not dependent, directly or indirectly, on the activity of all other elements of the same piece of gray substance.

Thus the cerebral cortex, the largest of the connected pieces of gray matter, may be responsible for the decisions that involve the most circumspect consideration of all the available data, i.e., of all the input that reaches the cortex. This is most of the input that reaches the brain, since even where sensory channels are connected directly to regions of the nervous system that organize the motor response, such as in the spinal cord or in the optic tectum, a copy of the input is relayed to the cerebral cortex for more general reference in the context of the global, multisensory experience.

▶

FIGURE 8.1. Transverse section through the right hemisphere of a human brain. The cortex covers the entire hemisphere as a folded band (*C*) stained more lightly than the underlying white substance (*M*). Within the cortex, especially in the upper regions of the hemisphere, a more superficial layer can be distinguished from a deeper layer, which is rich in intracortical myelinated fibers (B-system in our terminology) and therefore stains more darkly. The large fiber mass of the white substance (*M*) is composed mainly of the corticocortical fibers of the A-system. Some subcortical structures are also shown: *N:* head of the caudate nucleus, *S:* putamen; *P:* pallidum. Myelin stain. × 2

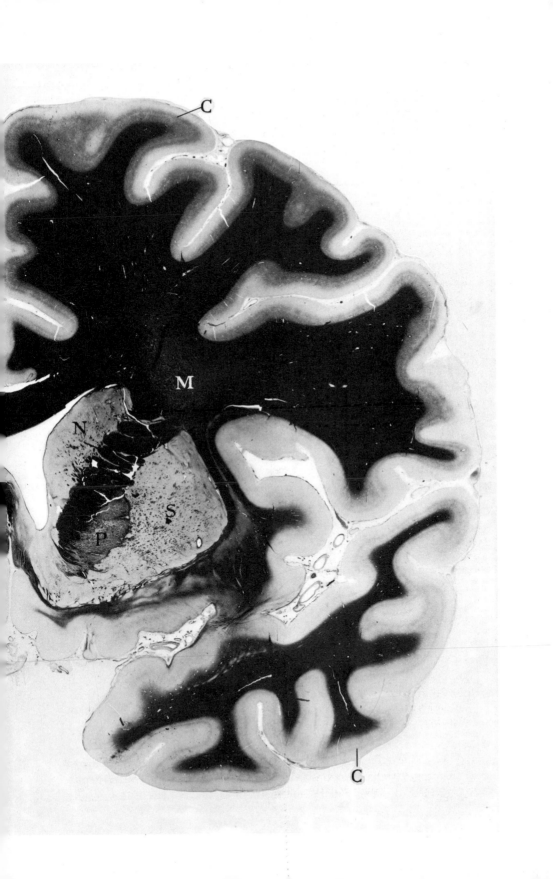

The fact that we have not one, but two cerebral cortices has been given much attention in recent years. The relation of the two, right and left, cortices is a very complicated one. There is ample evidence for the observation that the two cortices simply deal with the two halves of the world, the right cortex with everything that happens to the left of the plane of my nose, the left cortex vice versa. However, there are other experimental situations in which it seems that corresponding places of the right and left cortex are occupied with the same functions, as if one was simply there to check on the other or to replace the other in case of failure. Finally, there is more and more evidence indicating that many performances of the cortex simply disregard the anatomical bilateral symmetry and divide between themselves the available space, as if the cortex were equally suited everywhere to accommodate whatever needs are felt. This is particularly true for the storing of learned information: language mainly on the left, information about spatial structures on the right, etc. [8.9, 8.19].

2. The *type of symmetry* of the cortical nerve net has already been mentioned in connection with the cerebellum (Chapt. 6; Fig. 6.2). The cortex is a plate of fairly uniform thickness, covering most of the anterior part of the brain. While the fiber connections within the cortex are distributed uniformly in all directions of the cortical plane, so that vertical sections through the cortex look the same no matter how they are oriented, the up–down direction is markedly asymmetric. Very different types of fibers run in the two opposite directions, and most neurons of the cortex show a definite functional and morphologic polarization in the vertical direction.

The anatomical symmetry, suggesting homogeneous functional relations between the elements within the cortical plane, is in contrast with a popular view of the cortex as composed of sensory, motor, and associational regions. We usually imagine the information as reaching the cortex within the sensory regions, traversing the associational regions horizontally, and finally leaving again through the fiber tracts that originate in the motor cortex. It is astonishing that within the associational regions the direction of information flow does not correspond to any special set of fibers, which one might expect as the anatomical equivalent of the functional asymmetry implied by the terms input and output. Following the main tendency of this book, we shall take the anatomical situation seriously and try to reinterpret what we have learned from the physiologists in order to make their results fit the unquestionable propositions of anatomy. From this point of view, at this stage, we gain the following picture of the cortex. The vertically asymmetric organization of the cortical tissue, which is essentially similar throughout the cortical plane, corresponds to the fundamental operation that the cerebral cortex performs on its input. This should be an operation between layers, with one or more layers of the cortex serving as input stations and other layers as output. The main puzzle is the very similar structure of the cortex in motor, sensory, and other regions. The fundamental operation must be a very generally applicable one, if it is to make any sense in the context of visual, auditory, tactile, and olfactory information, in the organization of movements, in the perception and generation of speech, etc.

Before we turn to the fine structure of the connections within the cortex, there are some more remarks to be made on the macroscopic layout of the cortical tissue. Like the cerebellar cortex, it is folded in larger animals. The explanation is the same: if the fundamental operation is connected to a certain vertical organization, an increase in the volume of the cortex can only be achieved by an increase of its surface area. Such an increase may become necessary in larger animals because of the greater demands on informational space that their larger bodies and their larger environments pose. If the demand increases more than proportionally to the surface, say, proportionally to the volume of the animal, the cortex will have to be wrinkled. We have already mentioned that, at variance with the cerebellum, the behavior of the layers in the folding suggests that only neighborhood relations, not distances between the elements are preserved.

Comparative anatomy, and particularly, the position of the cerebral cortex in the immediate neighborhood of the olfactory bulbs suggests that in evolutionary history the origins of the cortex are connected with the sense of smell. It is curious that the olfactory input is unique in its relation to the cortex in two ways. Firstly, it is uncrossed, so that olfactory signals from the left nostril will be relayed mainly to the left hemisphere, contrary to the general crossed representation of the two halves of the world in the brain. Secondly, olfactory fibers enter the cortex from the surface, while all other fiber connections of the cerebral cortex are collected in the mass of the white substance underlying the cortex.

3. From its original role as a secondary or tertiary olfactory center, the cerebral cortex has developed into a central computing apparatus that is about equidistant, synaptically speaking, from all sensory neurons and from the neurons commanding the motor output. Not every neuron in the cortex, however, is only three or four synaptic steps removed from the sense cells and the motoneurons. Actually the vast majority of them cannot be directly associated with any of the input or output channels. We must think of them in a more abstract

way than as of a system of sensory and motor "projection," as was the fashion among the neurologists of the last century.

In fact, if we call output fibers all the fibers that leave the cortex and input fibers all the fibers that enter it, we obtain a very different picture. Most of the neurons of the cortex, as we shall see, have axons that leave the cortical gray substance. Thus the number of output fibers is of the same order as that of the cortical neurons, 10^{10} in man (10^7 in the mouse). The majority of these again enter the cortex after having traveled through the white substance, so that the number of input fibers is again of the same order of magnitude. If we compare to this the number of fibers in the sensory channels, which in man hardly exceeds the order of 10^6, we realize that most of the work the cortex does is on information that it itself provides. It seems that the cortex acts mainly and essentially in a *reflexive mode*. We are not surprised about this since it is intuitively obvious (and confirmed by many observations of experimental psychology) that our perceptions are always a mixture of a little input from the sensory channels with abundant information already present in memory. It is very difficult in particular situations to distinguish sensation from imagination, as everybody realizes when he is asked detailed questions about his experiences (e. g., as a witness in court), and the critical observer will have noticed that usually expectation prevails over immediate sensation.

If anybody objects that the relatively small number of external input fibers to the cortex, a few times 10^6, compared to the large number of corticocortical connections, refers only to the so-called specific afferents, while there are many more, so-called aspecific afferents to the cortex, he is only partially right. Most of these external afferents come via thalamic relay neurons. The number of cells in the thalamus, however, is by about two orders of magnitude smaller than the number of cells in the cortex both in the mouse and in man, so that it can still safely be said that the reflexive, corticocortical input is about hundred times as powerful as the entire external input to the cortex.

4. *Types of neurons.* If only the cell bodies and nuclei are stained, the cortex, excepting the uppermost 1/10 of its thickness appears almost uniformly populated with neural cell bodies. There are about

▶

FIGURE 8.2. From a Golgi preparation of the cerebral cortex of the mouse. The cell bodies of four pyramidal cells are shown, only one sharply in focus. Their basal dendrites, densely covered with spines and the collaterals of their descending axons form the B-system of our terminology. Up in the cortex is to the left in the picture

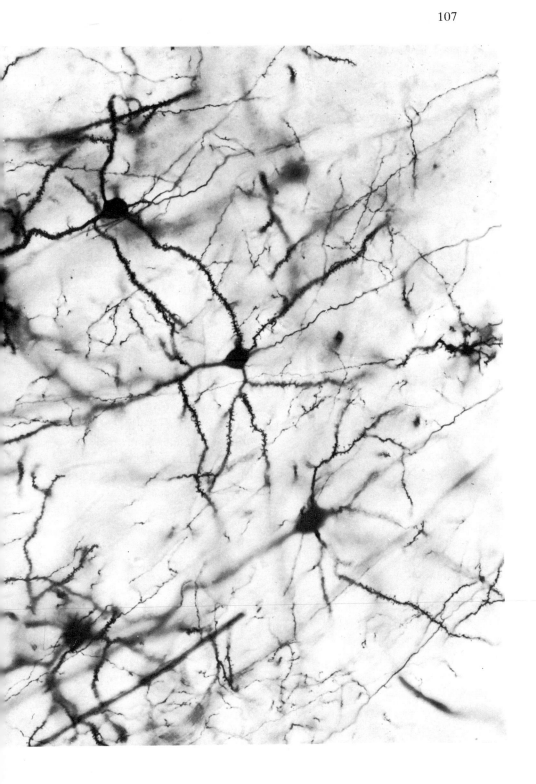

30,000 of them in one cubic millimeter of the human cortex, and about 200,000 in the mouse. The Golgi stain reveals a multitude of long and complicated dendritic and axonal cell-processes.

Cajal [8.6] and other neuroanatomists before and after him (e.g., Ref. [8.20]) have illustrated a great variety of shapes of cortical neurons, depending not only on the animal examined but also on the location of the specimen within the cortex and to a certain extent probably on sheer random variation from one neuron to the next. This variety has sometimes been quoted as an insurmountable difficulty in the analysis of the cerebral cortex and as an indication of a complexity that perhaps surpasses the limits of our understanding. I take the contrary stand and claim that the number of neural types in the cortex is very small, much smaller than, say, in the second ganglion, the medulla ganglionaris, of the fly, even if each type in the cortex undergoes some remarkable variations that may alter the relative and absolute size of its various components (cell body, dendrites, axons etc.) without changing the basic scheme of the connections. There are three main types of neurons in the cortex.

a) Pyramidal cells (Fig. 8.2). The following definition covers an estimated 75% of all cortical neurons. The dendritic tree is composed of two distinct portions. One, the apical dendrite, ramifies in the first (the uppermost) layer of the cortex. The other dendrites, the so-called basal dendrites, are distributed in roughly spherical symmetry around the cell body. The cell body may be located at all levels of the cerebral cortex, excepting the first, or molecular layer, making the distance between the apical and basal ramifications very different for different pyramidal cells of the same region of the cortex. The axonal tree is also composed of two parts. The first branches, the so-called axon collaterals, stay entirely within the cortex, usually occupying a region a little below and overlapping that of the basal dendrites. The main axon, which leaves the cell body in a downward direction, leaves the cortex and in almost all cases reenters it in a different place, where it ascends to the upper layer of the cortex and there splits up into terminal arborizations. Some of the main axons − or branches thereof − reach other places of the brain and thus constitute "output lines" in the narrower sense.

The dendrites of the pyramidal cells are studded with tiny spines, a few thousand for each neuron. This the pyramidal cells have in common with many other neurons, e.g., with the Purkinje cells of the cerebellum.

b) Martinotti cells. These are, in a way, antipodic to the pyramidal cells. Their cell bodies and dendrites lie in the lower layers of the cortex. Their axons ascend to the uppermost layer, the molecular layer, where the apical dendrites of all the pyramidal cells congregate, and there form long branches.

c) Stellate cells. Many neurons in the cortex are of a type that is widespread in the most diverse pieces of gray substance. The dendrites radiate in all directions around the cell body, justifying the name, while the axon breaks up into terminal ramifications within a region in the immediate vicinity, often generously overlapping the region of the dendrites. Depending on the shape and orientation of the axonal tree of stellate cells, a number of categories can be distinguished. However, since we do not know the meaning of these variations, we may disregard them for the time being and use the common characteristics of stellate cells as the definition of a third type of cortical neurons, well distinguished from pyramidal and Martinotti cells.

In addition to the shape of their dendritic and axonal trees, there are some other characteristics that justify the distinction of different types of neurons in the cortex. Thus spines are found only on the dendrites of pyramidal cells in any significant number. Although spiny stellate cells have occasionally been described, they must be considerably rarer than the usual types of stellate cells, which have smooth dendrites. Another striking distinction can be made on the basis of the density of the intracortical axonal ramification. Stellate cells have by far the densest axonal trees, while the axon collaterals of pyramidal cells are distributed over the widest regions and thus form the loosest ramification. Martinotti cells are in between in this respect [8.5].

5. A skeleton cortex. Pyramidal cells are so characteristic for the cerebral cortex, that on the basis of their presence, any small piece of cortical tissue can immediately and unequivocally be recognized as such. They are also numerically prevalent, as we have already said, and certainly make by far the largest contribution to the volume of the cortical gray substance. We are justified, therefore, in considering the set of all the pyramidal cells with their connections as the skeleton of the cortex and taking this as a basis for a functional model to which we may later add the other components as modifiers of the fundamental operation (Fig. 8.3).

Pyramidal cells are coupled together by two distinct systems of fiber connections. Every pyramidal cell partakes in the two systems. The two parts of the dendritic tree, apical and basal, and the two sets of axonal ramifications, main axon and axon collaterals, are the anatomical expression of this twofold coupling.

A-system: The apical dendrite of each pyramidal cell has abundant branches in the first (or molecular) layer, where it receives afferents from other pyramidal cells situated in more or less distant regions of the cortex. In turn, each pyramidal cell contributes axonal terminations to the molecular layer in some other cortical region.

B-system: The basal dendrites of each pyramidal cell are connected to the axon collaterals of nearby pyramidal cells.

Since the longest connections, spanning the whole extent of the cortex, are in the A-system, while the fibers of the B-system bridge at most a few millimeters (in man), the two systems could also be called long- and short-range systems, respectively. However, this distinction may in fact miss the point, which is that the probability of a B-connection between two cells is dependent on their distance in the cortex, while the probability of a direct link in the A-system may, for all we know, be independent of their relative positions or, at least, is not simply a monotonic function of their distance. Thus the terms metrically dependent, or for short, *metric connections* for the B-system and not metrically dependent, or *ametric connections* for the A-system may be more appropriate [8.16].

Judging from the relative size of the apical and basal dendrites, the amount of coupling in the two systems is about the same. We may conclude from this that each pyramidal cell is as much under the influence of its neighbors within its own area as it is under the influence of activity spread over the entire cortex.

The distinction between the A- and B-systems of pyramidal cell connections is further made interesting because of the different symmetries of the two systems. While we have no reason to suppose that in the long-range or A-system the probability of a certain pyramidal cell sending a fiber toward another pyramidal cell should not be the same as that of a fiber running in the opposite direction, the situation is different in the B-system. In fact the axon collaterals of pyramidal cells tend to be distributed in a layer below that of the basal dendrites of the same cell, so that the probability of an axon–collateral–basal dendrite connection is much higher in the direction from a cell in

▶

FIGURE 8.3. The skeleton cortex, composed only of pyramidal cells. There are some exceptional regions: *O*, the olfactory cortex, where the afferent fibers enter the uppermost layer, *M*, the motor cortex, which sends output fibers to the motor periphery of the nervous system and *S*, the primary sensory areas that receive a special set of afferent fibers. The general case is the cortex with long-range, ametric, subcortical connections and with short-range, metrically dependent, intracortical connections (A and B systems in our terminology). *B*: axon collaterals forming the B-system. *C*: convergence of fibers from the whole cortex onto a small region (A-system)

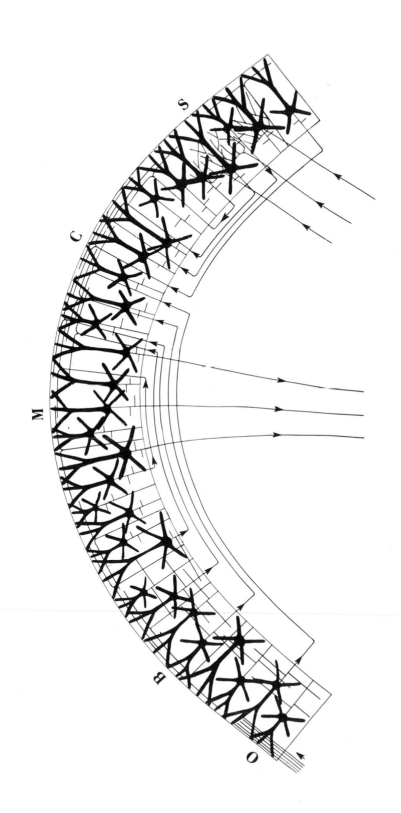

a higher layer toward a cell in a lower layer than vice versa. Thus we have more opportunity for symmetric, reciprocal connections in the A-system and more opportunity for cascaded, irreciprocal connections in the vertical direction in the B-system.

This observation makes it even more interesting that in some parts of the cortex, in the so-called allocortex, the pyramidal cells tend to be aligned in one layer. There the opportunity for unidirectional chains of connections in the B-system is sacrificed in favor of a denser net of reciprocal connections. The fact comes to mind that the hippo-campus, one of the regions where this is true, is particularly prone to generate seizure activity, i. e., easily reaches a state where the neurons excite each other to a paroxism of synchronous activity.

The ability to sustain seizure activity both locally and over the whole cortex requires a vast net of excitatory connections. Actually, since diffuse stimulation of the cortex, e. g., by electric currents, pre-sumably activates excitatory as well as inhibitory neurons but regular-ly leads to a seizure, we must conclude that the excitatory connections override the inhibitory ones, the latter not being able to check the increase of activity once a certain density of active neurons has been reached. It is tempting then to conclude that the pyramidal cells, which furnish the bulk of the short- and long-range connections, are excitatory in nature. While there is some incertitude among neuro-physiologists about this point, I will simply assume that the skeleton cortex contains only excitatory synapses. The system of pyramidal cells with their double sets of connections is then essentially a device that allows self-sustained activity (of which the epileptic seizure is an exaggerated caricature!) in ensembles of coupled neurons. The addi-tional neurons, and especially the stellate cells, which are frequently suspected of being inhibitory, may then form a necessary complemen-tary mechanism that prevents the extension of the activity beyond the desired level.

6. *Some quantitative considerations.* Before we set out to invent some plausible uses for this vast system of coupled neurons, let us look more closely at the quantities involved.

We may ask, for instance, whether the idea of every place of the cortex sending fibers to and receiving fibers from every other place is at all compatible with the observed volume of the white substance. A crude estimate can be obtained as follows. If a round flat surface is subdivided into many compartments and if each compartment is con-nected to each of the others by a straight line, the average length of the connecting line segments, according to my colleague Dr. G. Palm, is $(16/3\pi - 8/9)r$, a little less than the radius r of the round surface. If the surface is convex, like the cortex of the mouse or even more like that of man, and if the connections may take the most direct routes, the average length is a little less but may still be of the same order. If we know the number of pyramidal cells and if we suppose that the axon of each of them makes a corticocortical connection, the volume of the resulting mass of white substance is easily calculated by multiplying this number by the average length and average cross section of the fibers. It turns out that the volume of the hemispheric white substance in the mouse as well as in man is close to the calculated value. The idea of a complete set of point to point connections, independent of the distance, as the term ametric system implies, is at least compatible with the gross anatomy.

The next question is, how large would the compartments of the cortex have to be so that it could be said that each is connected to each of the others? Evidently, if they are too small, they will not contain enough pyramidal cells to provide the axons for each of the other compartments, since each pyramidal cell probably gives off only one corticocortical fiber. From this point of view, a convenient parceling of the cortex would be such that the resulting compartments contain as many pyramidal cells as there are such compartments. This would make the number of compartments and the number of cells in each compartment equal to the square root of the total number of pyramidal cells. Such compartments in the cortex of man would have a diameter of about 1 mm, in the mouse about 0.17 mm. It is noteworthy that both in man and in the mouse this size corresponds to the dendritic spread of the largest pyramidal cells. If our idea of a diffuse distribution of the fibers in the A-system is correct, each compartment may contain information about the state of the rest of the cortex. Thus each large pyramidal cell may receive through its apical dendrite a global picture of the activity of the entire cortex.

Of course, to receive just one fiber out of every compartment would not be any significant information about the state of the cortex, unless within each compartment the activities of individual cells were strongly correlated. We may take the discovery of so-called columns containing neurons with uniform characteristics [8.11, 8.15] as an indication that this is indeed so.

A quantitative look at the fibers of the B-system also has some surprises for us. Each pyramidal cell (in the mouse) produces about 4 to 6 mm of intracortical axon collaterals (Fig. 8.2). If we multiply this value by the number of pyramidal cells, it turns out that this is the most substantial contribution to the intracortical axonal felt: at least half of the 1.2 km of axonal fibers that are contained in every cubic millimeter of the mouse cortex. It is interesting to compare the total length of the axonal felt with the number of synapses contained in one cubic mm of cortex, which is nearly 10^9 in the mouse [8.7]. If 10^9 μm of axon are presynaptic to 10^9 synapses, there must be on an average one synapse every μm of axonal length. The axon collaterals of the pyramidal cells find their way through the dense feltwork of the dendrites of neighboring pyramidal cells, making thousands of synaptic contacts along their way. The axon collaterals of pyramidal cells are peculiarly straight, much straighter, say, than the collaterals of the ascending Martinotti cell axons or of the afferent fibers to the cortex. This has an interesting consequence. It is not likely that an axon collateral meets a particular dendritic tree of another pyramidal cell more than once on its straight course through the network, about as unlikely as it is to hit a tree twice with a bullet shot through its (leafless) crown. The connections in the B-system seem to be arranged in such a way as to guarantee the distribution of signals from one neuron onto the largest possible number of other neurons and, of course, vice versa, the greatest possible convergence from many neighbors onto one target cell. The factor of convergence–divergence, in the B-system of the mouse, is at least 1000, more likely 2000. Presumably the convergence is about the same in the A-system.

Altogether we arrive at the picture of the cortex as a gigantic mixing machine. Every small bit of the cortical gray substance contains information about the state of a very large number of cortical cells. There are clearly two sets of neurons that project their information onto any one small region: the neighbors within a radius of at most a few millimeters that reach it through the B-system, and a set of cells distributed throughout the whole cortex (in reality even throughout both, right and left, cortices), which contribute their axons through the A-system. The holographic analogy, which has been in fashion lately, is correct in this sense: the macroscopic distribution of activity in the cortex is projected everywhere onto small regions of the cortex itself. This explains some of the plasticity that has been observed following lesions of the cortex. Loss of cortical substance in delimited regions does not in general abolish certain well-defined competences of the cortex, but rather produces a general impairment of function, just as a partial destruction of the hologram reduces the amount of information about the picture represented, but does not lead to the loss of any part of it.

7. *Feature detectors and cell assemblies.* Although the last word has not yet been said, it seems that individual neurons of the cortex do not represent complicated situations, such as the "things" and

"events" of our psychological experience, but much simpler properties of the input for which the term "features" is often used. Neurons in the visual cortex tend to be "feature detectors" for the visual input, the neurons in the auditory or somatosensory cortex detect similar elementary features of the auditory or tactile input. Even if many neurons within and outside the sensory areas of the cortex respond to features in more than one sensory modality, they do not seem to represent by their activity an organized whole of a complexity approaching that of the perception of another animal, or a tree, or of a spoken sentence, or even word. In the visual system these features have been extensively studied (especially by Hubel and Wiesel) and do not seem to go much beyond such definitions as "white spot surrounded by shadow in a certain region of the visual field" or "a transition from light to dark, with a boundary oriented at 45°, somewhere in a certain region of the visual field." Even outside of the sensory regions the language of individual neurons remains fairly simple. Thus fibers of the corpus callosum, which are sensitive to visual input, seem to respond also to the sort of properties that excite the neurons in the visual areas [8.2]. Since the corpus callosum belongs to the A-system of our terminology, this finding would imply that the internal communications of the cortex also do not make use of any more complicated code in single neurons.

The inference that can be drawn from this is that the relevant "things" of our experience are represented within the brain not by single neurons but by sets of neurons. Just how many neurons are involved in the internal image of a thing like "my house" or "the neighbor's dog" or "the tune of Greensleeves" is very difficult to say, but it is likely that their number is too large for any neurophysiologist ever to be able to record their activity by multiple-electrode recording. The sets of neurons that stand for certain events, or objects of the outside world, the "cell assemblies" as they were called by Hebb [8.2], must have a certain internal coherence, since it is one of the basic observations of psychology that partial evidence of a thing tends to make us perceive the whole thing. This is best explained by supposing that the elements of a cell assembly are coupled by excitatory synapses, so that the excitation of some of them ignites the whole set and leaves all of them in a state of excitation until their activity is again extinguished by external inhibition. If we want to localize cell assemblies more concretely in the cortex, we notice that they are of two sorts — restricted to particular areas, or diffuse. The cell assembly "my neighbor's dog" represents within my brain a very complicated bundle of properties in various sensory modalities and must occupy almost the entire cortex. On the other hand, the cell assembly "Greensleeves" may be localized in the auditory region of the brain and may indeed persist undisturbed by any other activity my cortex may be involved in.

Some more properties of cell assemblies come to mind. Some are essentially synchronous, like motionless visual images, others have a temporal structure, like the cell assembly representing Greensleeves. The synchronous ones are composed of parts any one of which may recall the others, while the asynchronous ones lack this symmetry, since obviously it is much easier to recall the tune of Greensleeves starting from the beginning than from the end. However, some temporal structures, such as the words of a language, seem to be represented almost in a synchronous way, since it is about as easy to find words that rhyme with a given word as it is to find words beginning with the same letters: the asynchronous cell assemblies representing the words can be activated in the direction of time as well as in the opposite direction.

It is likely that the neural connections holding the cell assemblies together are provided by the fibers that interconnect sets of cortical pyramidal cells. The fibers of the A-system would then be responsible for the diffuse complex cell assemblies, while the B-system would be involved mainly in localized cell assemblies. We have already noted that the A-system is essentially symmetric and so are the associations that bind the various properties of "my neighbor's dog." On the contrary, the connections between axon collaterals and basal dendrites are more directional in the sense that the downward direction is favored. It is tempting to make the vertical direction in the B-system responsible for the temporal structure of some localized cell assemblies.

8. *Learning.* Clearly, cell assemblies representing particular people, musical tunes, or words of a language cannot be genetically predetermined. They must arise by a process of learning. The connections between pyramidal cells must develop as a consequence of experience, or must be modifiable by experience according to certain laws. The simplest idea, the oldest and probably the best, is that correlation in time of the activity of two or more neurons leads to these neurons becoming connected by excitatory synapses. In a crude way, the neurophysiology of learning has long been established. If electric stimuli to the motor cortex that elicit movement, are paired with electric stimuli to the visual cortex, after a while stimulation of the visual cortex will be sufficient by itself to make the animals perform just those movements that previously occurred only after stimulation of the motor area [8.1, 8.8, 8.14]. Here correlation of activity leads to new connec-

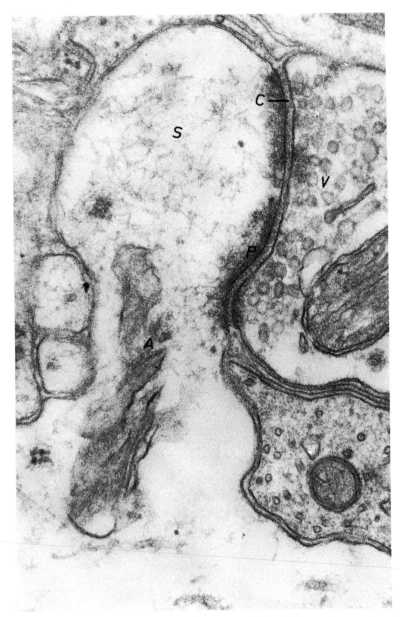

FIGURE 8.4. Dendritic spine of a pyramidal cell from the cortex of the mouse. Compare spines in the Golgi pictures (Figs. 4.2, 4.3, and 8.2) at lower magnification. Except for the synaptic vesicles (*V*), the structural details around the synapse are poorly understood in functional terms: *C:* synaptic cleft; *P:* postsynaptic density; *A:* spine apparatus. The growth of spines or modifications of their fine structure have sometimes been considered as the possible substrate of memory. Electron micrograph, × 90,000

tions in the cortex, but the effect is macroscopic and difficult to interpret. More recently, changes in the pattern of connections of single cells of the cerebral cortex have been demonstrated in various instances. The most convincing observation [8.12] refers to the cells of the visual cortex of the cat, which receive input from corresponding places of the two retinae. We must suppose that the cortical cells discover in the surrounding fiber felt those afferents that have correlated (i.e., practically identical) activities because they relay information from parallel lines of sight in the two eyes, and that they establish synapses with just such correlated sets of fibers. In fact, if the correlation is disrupted during the critical learning phase, e.g., by masking the two eyes in alternation, so that they can never present their input at the same time to the cerebral cortex, most cortical cells will later be found to have only or predominantly monocular connections. This is exactly what theorists have been expecting for the longest time: connections between individual elements of the nervous system being established on the basis of statistical correlations in their activity.

The anatomy of learning has stayed far behind theory and electrophysiology. We do not know whether the changes are in the pattern of axonal connections, or whether the dendrites or dendritic spines (Fig. 8.4) are the modifiable elements [8.18]. Possibly the changes in the structure of the net are even more subtle and perhaps invisible in the microscope. The modification of the strength of the coupling in an already existing synapse may escape the resolution of the electron microscope. Quite likely, however, ontogenetic memory is laid down in the same form as genetic memory, namely, in the variation of the shape of neuronal ramifications. It may escape microscopic observation not because the structures involved are too small, but because they are embedded in a net of unmanageable complexity. We notice the difficulty when we subject animals to "artificial environments" in the hope of later discovering in the brain the artificially induced memory traces. Either the artificial environment is so brutally disruptive that the effect could hardly be compared to ordinary learning, or, if we stay within the physiologic range and induce more gentle engrams, we do not know where to look for them.

9. *Input, output, and additional equipment.* I have emphasized the internal connections of the cortex, rather than the input and output connections, because of their sheer bulk and also because there is a tendency elsewhere to describe the cortex just as an additional way station in the sensory channels, an additional layer of the retina or of the lateral and medial geniculate nuclei. The rich connections between pyramidal cells and, especially, the connections between the various

sensory channels are undoubtedly the most impressive feature of the cortical level. However, they would be of no use unless their network were fed initially and later continually prompted by information from the senses. The relation of the sensory afferents, relayed through the thalamus, and the system of pyramidal cells is not clear even to the electrophysiologists who specifically study this problem. It seems, however, that the sensory input has fairly direct access to some of the pyramidal cells since the feature detectors whose activity has been observed in direct correlation with sensory events, are for the most part pyramidal cells [8.21]. In some cases there may be a stellate cell, a so-called interneuron, interposed between the sensory fiber and the pyramidal cell, perhaps for the purpose of switching an excitatory signal to an inhibitory one. This is in accordance with the observation that small stellate cells populate particularly the sensory areas of the cortex and are especially frequent at the layer of the cortex, the so-called fourth layer, where the thalamic afferent fibers terminate.

The output poses no problem. A representative sample of cortical pyramidal cells has axons that reach various levels of the motor system. Some, certainly a minority, have direct access to the "final common path," the motoneuron innervating the muscle.

What is still very obscure is the relation of the cortex to all the additional equipment to which it is connected. If the cortex is nothing but a mixer of information for the purpose of discovering and recording correlated activity, there must be various control units in order to make good use of this. There must be an insurance against the seizure-like explosion of the cortical activity, probably by feedback onto the thresholds of cortical neurons. If cell-assemblies are the terms of the cortical logic, there must be a device for the discovery of the ignition of a cell assembly and there must be the possibility of extinguishing cell assemblies. There must be a timer that regulates the succession of activated cell assemblies. There must also be a mechanism of attention that inhibits entire regions of the cortex once something interesting has ignited somewhere. Finally, there must be mechanisms that connect the rather cool cortical memory by correlation with the more impassioned system of inborn patterns of behavior, which is also subject to learning of some sort. It would be tempting to identify these postulated mechanisms with particular anatomical locations, but I prefer to continue my speculations on a more abstract level.

10. *Macrocosm and microcosm.* Insufficient as this picture of the cortex may be, it is close to a philosophical paradigm, that of the order of the external world mirrored in the internal structure of the individual. If synapses are established between neurons as a conse-

quence of their synchronous activation, the correlations between the external events represented by these neurons will be translated into correlations of their activity that will persist independently of further experience. The synaptic structure of the nerve net will approximate the causal structure of the environment.

The image of the world in our brain is an expression that should not be understood in an all too pictorial, geometric sense. True, there are many regions in the brain where the coordinates of the nerve tissue directly represent the coordinates of some sensory space, as in the primary visual area of the cortex or in the acoustic centers. But in many other instances we should rather think of the image in the brain as of a graph representing the transition probabilities between situations mirrored in the synaptic relations between neurons. Also, it is not my environment that is photographed in my brain, but the environment plus myself, with all my actions and perceptions smoothly integrated in my internal representation of the world. I can experience how fluid the border between myself and my environment is when I scratch the surface of a stone with a stick and localize the sensation of roughness in the tip of the stick, or when I have to localize my consciousness in the rear of my car in order to back it into a narrow parking space.

11. Prediction. The image of the world in the brain is a dynamic representation; not only the neighborhood relations and other forms of association of things are represented, but also the laws that govern the evolution of the environment. The patterns of activity within the brain that represent the present state continually go over into new patterns even if the sensory channels are temporarily closed, by virtue of the internal synaptic connections. If the brain is well wired, this evolution of the internal state matches the evolution that would be otherwise imposed by the changes of the input. Thus the capacity to predict the future is an essential attribute of the brain.

Normally, in the process that we call perception, the sensory input and the internal prediction are inextricably mixed. They are the two irreducible components of the process of acquisition of knowledge in all cases where the available information is incomplete. And the amount of information is always insufficient as long as the brain is so small and the world so large. In science these two components are called hypothesis and experiment.

As in science, so also in the brain the discrepancy between the prediction and the actual evolution of the input is used continually to amend the predicting mechanism. Not only a new hypothesis has to be developed, when the old one proves wrong, but the principles that generate the hypotheses have to be revised. This is how the information from the macrocosm is incorporated into the microcosm of the brain.

The brain as a foretelling machine clashes with the more down to earth view of the brain as an input-output device that gives appropriate responses to sensory stimuli. However, the two views can be reconciled. The prediction that the brain makes at all times by letting its internal state evolve in accordance with the most probable evolution of the world, contains also a prediction of the future position of the animal itself within its environment. We may suppose that the motor output secondarily follows the prediction of the next state of the motor system. In the action of tracking a moving object we notice how our output is not governed by the immediate input but is, rather, a consequence of an ongoing prediction. When we sing in unison with other singers, we notice the curious ambiguity between action and perception. Subjectively one's own action of singing is perceived in a smooth blend with the singing of the others, or both seem to emerge from a continual process of prediction. We are reminded of the anatomy of the cortex where the motor area is not subordinated to the sensory areas, but arranged in parallel with them in the continuum of the cortical plane.

12. The Principle of Optimism. To predict one's own motor output makes sense only if the predicting mechanism has a bias toward the more advantageous developments. Only then, if the next state of the world as predicted by the brain will bring some changes for the better, will it be useful to make the adjustments of the motor system implied by the prediction.

But how does the optimism get into the brain? It seems to me that this is simply a consequence of natural selection and of the ability of the predictor to learn. Suppose that for a given input two different predictions were possible, one favorable and the other catastrophic. A pessimistic brain chooses the gloomy prediction. If the prediction was correct, it is automatically eliminated. If it was incorrect, it survives but the predicting mechanism will be amended to make it less pessimistic. Consider, on the contrary, an optimistic brain that tends to predict the favorable alternative. If the future proves it to be right, there is no need for a correction. If it was wrong, there is no chance for one. Altogether optimism will prevail.

References

8.1   Baer, A.: Über gleichzeitige elektrische Reizung zweier Großhirnstellen am ungehemmten Hunde. Pflügers Arch. Ges. Physiol. *106*, 523–67 (1905)

8.2 Berlucchi, G., Gazzaniga, M.S., Rizzolatti, G.: Microelectrode analysis of transfer of visual information by the corpus callosum of cat. Arch. Ital. Biol. *105*, 583–596 (1967)

8.3 Braitenberg, V.: Thoughts on the Cerebral Cortex. J. Theor. Biol. *46*, 421–447 (1974)

8.4 Braitenberg, V.: On the representation of objects and their relations in the brain. In: Lecture Notes in Biomathematics. 4. Physics and Mathematics of the Nervous System, Conrad, M., Güttinger, W., Dal Cin, M. (eds.) Berlin–Heidelberg–New York: Springer, 1974, pp. 290–298

8.5 Braitenberg, V.: Cortical Architectonics, General and Areal. In: Architectonics of the Cerebral Cortex. M.A.B. Brazier and H. Petsche, eds. New York: Raven Press 1977. pp. 443–465

8.6 Cajal, S.R.: Histologie du système nerveux de l'homme et des vertébrés. Paris: Maloin 1911

8.7 Cragg, B.G.: The density of synapses and neurones in the motor and visual areas of the cerebral cortex. J. Anat. *101*, 4, 639–654 (1967)

8.8 Doty, R.W.: Conditioned Reflexes elicited by Electrical Stimulation of the Brain in Macaques. J. Neurophysiol. *28*, 623–640 (1965)

8.9 Gazzaniga, M.S.: The Bisected Brain. Neuroscience Series, Vol. II Towe, A. (ed.), New York: Meredith Corp., 1970

8.10 Hebb, D.O.: The Organization of Behaviour. New York: Wiley, 1949

8.11 Hubel, D.H., Wiesel, T.N.: Receptive fields, binocular interaction and functional architecture in the cat's visual cortex. J. Physiol. *160*, 106 (1962)

8.12 Hubel, D.H., Wiesel, T.N.: Receptive fields and function architectonics in two non-striate visual areas (18 and 19) of the cat. J. Neurophysiol. *28*, 229–289 (1965)

8.13 Hume, D.: A Treatise of Human Nature (London 1738), London: Dent, 1961

8.14 Loucks, R.B.: Preliminary report of a technique for stimulation or destruction of tissues beneath the integument and the establishing of conditioned reactions with faradization of the cerebral cortex. J. Comp. Psychol. *16*, 439–444 (1933)

8.15 Mountcastle, V.B.: Modality and topographic properties of single neurons of cat's somatic sensory cortex. J. Neurophysiol. *20*, 408 (1957)

8.16 Palm, G., Braitenberg, V.: Tentative contributions of neuroanatomy to nerve net theories. In: Symp. 3rd Europ. Meet. Cybernetics and Systems Research 1976. Trappl, R. (ed.) 1977 in press

8.17 Parmenides: In: Nahm, M.C.: Selections from Early Greek Philosophy. 4th ed. New York: Meredith Publ. Comp., 1964, p. 93

8.18 Schüz, A.: Some facts and hypotheses concerning dendritic spines and learning. In: Architectonics of the Cerebral Cortex. M.A.B. Brazier and H. Petsche, eds. New York: Raven Press 1977

8.19 Sperry, R.W.: Brain bisection and consciousness. In: Brain and Conscious Experience, Eccles, J.C. (ed.). New York: Springer 1966, pp. 298–313

8.20 Szentágothai, J.: Synaptology of the visual cortex. In: Handbook of Sensory Physiology, Vol. VII/3, Part B. R. Jung (ed.) New York, 1973

8.21 Van Essen, D., Kelly, J.: Correlation of cell shape and function in the visual cortex of the cat. Nature (London) *241*, 403–405 (1973)

Subject Index

A

abnormal wiring 56
acetic acid 28
acetylcholine 26, 27, 36
action potential 23
after-potential 23
alarm clock 75
alcohol 28
allocortex 112
ametric connections 110
amino acids 30
anatomical-physiologic dictionary
  36
anatomy 43
Anaxagoras 9
animism 4
aperture 46
apical dendrite 108
area 101
arthropods 62
artificial environment 118
aspecific afferents 106
associational region 104
asynchronous cell assemblies 116
A-system 109, 110
ataxia 77
axodendritic contact 36
axon 32, 34, 37
axonal ramification 32
axonal tree 32
axon-collateral-basal dendrite connection 110
axon collaterals of pyramidal cells
  108, 113, 114
axon hillock 34

B

basal dendrites 108
Beckett 1
behavior 83
bilateral symmetry 16
biology 8
bit 14
brain pathology 56
branches of the axon 32
B-system 110, 112, 113,
  114
butterfly 11

C

Cajal 108
cascaded connections 112
causality 77
cell assemblies 115, 116
cell body 32, 34, 37
cell membrane 21
cell nucleus 32, 37
celloidin 28
cerebellar cortex 64–78
cerebellar cortex as a clock 74
cerebellar map 72
cerebellar patients 78
cerebellar vermis 71
cerebellum 64
cerebral cortex 61, 66, 68, 72, 73,
  101
chance 41
changes in the synaptic pattern 43
channel capacity 10
chemical synapse 26, 27, 36

chloroform 28
clean slate 41
climbing fibers 69, 71, 75
coding 10
comparative anatomy 105
compartment 112, 113
complexity 37
compound eye 44, 84
computation 38
computer 2
concentration gradient 54
connective tissue 30
consciousness 4, 120
convergence 114
coordination of rapid movements
    76
corpus callosum 115
cortex 62
cortex, cerebellar 64–78
cortex, cerebral 101–119
cortex-like structure 43
cortical plane 66
cortices 62, 66
corticocortical connections 113
cross-correlation function 76
cybernetics 77
cyclostomes 78
crystals 5
crystals and texts 7

D

decrement 25, 39
decremental conduction 39
degeneration methods 30
delay line 76
dendrite 32, 34, 118
dendritic spine 34
dendritic tree 32, 34, 39
density of synapses in the cortex
    114
density of the intracortical axonal ra-
    mification 109
depolarization 25
dictionary 27
differential permeability for Na^+ and
    K^+ions 22
divergence 114
DNA 42
duality 40

E

electric coupling of neurons 76
electric synapse 25, 26, 36, 69
electrical interference of signals 38
electron microscope 21, 28, 34, 36
electrophysiology 2
electrotonic transmission 25
environment 11
environmental determination of
    brain structure 41
equator 54
equilibrium 72, 78
excitation 26
excitation level 39
excitatory synapse 36
explanation 7, 80

F

facet eye 44
family resemblance 59
feature detector 114, 115
feedback circuit 77, 78
fibrous structure 19
fish 78
fixation 28
fly 44
folding 62, 73
folding of cortex-like structures 70
form 84
formaldehyde 28
frequency modulation 39, 40
functional neuroanatomy 3
fuse 24

G

Galilei 83
gas 7
genetic determination of brain struc-
    ture 41
genetically determined information
    61
geometry 59, 60, 62, 66
glia 30
glia cell 20, 21
glutaraldehyde 28
Gnathonemus 64
Golgi method 30
Golgi stain 30, 108
gradient 54

granular cell 67, 69
granular layer 68, 73
gray matter 37, 38, 102
Griesinger 19

H

hardening 28
Hebb 115
Heisenberg 5
hemispheric white substance 113
hexagonal array of dots 52
hippocampus 112
histological techniques 27
histophysiologic dictionary 36
hologram 114
homogeneity 66
homology 62
homunculus 72
Horridge and Meinertzhagen 52
horseradish peroxydase 30
Hubel and Wiesel 115
Hume 101
hypothesis 80, 120

I

idea 84
image of the world in the brain 120
inborn structure 41
individual differences 60
inferior olive 69
information 9, 14
information capacity 10
information carrier 7
informational capacity of the genetic
    text 42
inhibition 27
inhibitory synapse 36
initial segment of the axon 39
input and output of the cortex 106
input to the cerebral cortex 102
insect brain 38
intention tremor 78
interpeduncular nucleus 71
intracortical axonal felt 113
invariants 60
invariants of cerebellar structure 64
invariant patterns 60
invertebrates 37

invertebrate brain 27
ion 22

K

Katz 19
K^+ ion 22
knowledge 15
Krafft-Ebing 19

L

lamina ganglionaris 43, 50, 54
landing maneuvers of the fly 87
language 5, 104, 116
learning 41, 43, 116
learning of correlations 118
local structural variations 61

M

macroscopic anatomy 3
macroscopic observation 5
many-neuron interaction 38
Martinotti cells 108, 109, 114
mechanism 4
medical schools 3
medulla ganglionaris 108
membrane potential 22, 23
memory 2, 8, 43, 118
memory traces 41
message 13, 14
metric connection 110
microelectrode 26
microelectrode recording 3
microcosm, macrocosm 11, 119
microscopic and macroscopic expla-
    nations 7
microtome 28
midline 71
mimicry 10
mirror symmetry 67
molecular layer 67, 73, 108, 109,
    110
mossy fibers 69, 71
motion perception 89
motoneuron 26, 27
motor cortex 104
movement detectors 85, 98
movement detectors, distribution
    91

movement detectors, multiplication
    92
movement detectors, orientation 95
movement detectors, spacing 89
myelin 20
myelin sheath 37
myelin stain 28
myelinated fibers 37

N

Na$^+$ion 22
neural types in the cortex 108
nerve cell membrane 21
nerve fiber 30
nerve tissue 19
nervous integration 38
neuroanatomical invariants 59
neuroanatomist 66
neuroanatomy 1
neuromuscular synapse 36
neuron 6, 39
neuronal membrane 22
neuro-ommatidium 50
neurophysiology 3
neuropil 38
Nissl stain 28
node of Ranvier 37
noise 59
number of fibers in the sensory chan-
    nels 106

O

olfactory bulbs 105
olfactory glomeruli 62
olfactory input to the cortex 105
olivary nucleus 76
ommatidium 46
optical resolution 44
optimism 121

P

paraffin 28
parallel fibers 67, 68, 69, 74
parallel folding 70
Parmenides 101
particle 5
perception 8, 120
permeability 27
permeability of the membrane 24

phase-shifted symmetric movement
    79
plasticity 114
positive feedback 24
potassium dichromate 28
potassium lock 23
prediction 13, 120, 121
principle of addressed communica-
    tion 20
probability 14
projection 38
projection of the visual field 52
proprioceptive feedback 78
proprioceptive system 77
pseudopupil 48
psychology 1, 83, 115
psychose 56
Purkinje cells 67, 68, 69, 73, 74,
    75, 108
pyramidal cells 108, 109, 112, 113,
    116

R

randomness 42
rapid movement 71, 78
reaction time 40
reciprocal interaction 54
redundancy 10, 17, 43
reflexive mode 106
refractoriness 39
resting potential 22
retina 10
retinula 46, 48, 50

S

seizure activity 112
sense organ 39
sensory afferents to the cortex 119
sensory regions of the cortex 104
set of transformations 60
shape of cortical neurons 108
shape of dendritic trees 34
silver 30
single-neuron physiology 38
skeleton cortex 109
sodium lock 23
sodium-potassium pump 22
sodium pump 22
source 12

source of information   12
specific afferent   106
speed of conduction   37
spike   23, 24, 26, 34, 36, 39
spike frequency   39
spike sequence   23, 39
spike transmission   37
spike-wave   24
spinal cord   26
spine   36, 108, 109, 118
staining techniques   28
stellate cells   109, 112, 119
stopwatch   75
structure   13
symmetry   59, 62, 72
symmetry of the cortex   104
synapse   25, 36, 37, 39, 54
synaptic cleft   36
synaptic transmitter substance   36
synaptic vesicle   36
syncytium   21
synthetic resin   28
systematic variation   59

T

tabula rasa   41
teleologic interpretation   80
teletype machine   11
television   9
text   5
textbook of anatomy   42
thalamic relay neurons   106
threshold   36, 39
threshold of the membrane potential   24

time   74
time-shifted pulse   79
timing   76
timing organ   74
topologic property   59
transformation and invariance   59
transmitter substance   26
tremor   77
types of neurons in the cortex   106
typical neuron   32

U

uncertainty   12
uniformity of the cerebellar operation   70
upright posture   71

V

velocity of conduction   37
vertebrates   37
vertebrate brain   27
vestibular nucleus   78
violin   76
visual ganglion   62, 97
visual ganglion of the fly   83
volume of the white substance   112

W

white-eyed fly   56
white-eyed mutant   54
white matter   37, 38
white substance   38, 106
Wiener   77
word   116

Studies of Brain Function

Editors: V. Braitenberg (Coordinating Editor),
H. B. Barlow, E. Florey, O.-J. Grüsser, H. van der Loos

Volume 1

W. HEILIGENBERG

Principles of Electrolocation and Jamming Avoidance in Electric Fish

A Neuroethological Approach

58 figures, 1 table. VI, 98 pages. 1977
ISBN 3-540-08367-7

Electric fish assess their environment by monitoring distortions of current fields generated by their own electric organ discharges. Much as echolocating bats, "electrolocating" fish orient themselves by evaluating feedback from their own action. Their performance may suffer as signals of different animals interfere and particular mechanisms have evolved to avoid mutual "jamming". Behavioral and neurophysiological data are presented to explain mechanisms of electrolocation and jamming avoidance, and the benefits of a parallel approach on behavioral and neuronal levels are demonstrated. The relative simplicity of natural stimuli and behaviors, of which some can even be elicted in neurophysiological preparations, renders electric fish a superb model system for neuroethological research.

Contents: General Physiological and Anatomical Background: The Electric Organ. Electroreceptors. Taxonomy of Electrolocating Fish. The Spectral Composition of Electric Organ Discharges. The Neuroanatomy of Electric Fish. – The Mechanism of Electrolocation: Spatial Aspects of Electrolocation. Response Characteristics and Central Projections of Tuberous Electroreceptors. Central Processing of Electric Images. Behavioral Measures of Electrolocation Performance. Electrolocation Performance in the Presence of Electric Noise and Mechanisms of Jamming Avoidance. Neuronal Mechanisms Linked to Jamming Avoidance and Electrolocation Under Jamming Conditions. Hypotheses and Results. Speculations on the Evolution of Pulse- and Water-type Electric Fish.

Springer-Verlag
Berlin
Heidelberg
New York

WITHDRAWN